The Anti-Aging Miracles of Hemp-Derived CBD Oil

The Anti-Aging Miracles of Hemp-Derived CBD Oil

• • •

5,000 Years of Healing The Body and The Brain

Sally Schutz, M.D. & Bayne Boyes, FCPA

© Copyright 2016 by Sally Schutz, M.D. & Bayne Boyes, FCPA
All rights reserved.

ISBN: 1519510802
ISBN 13: 9781519510808

This document is geared toward providing exact and reliable information in regard to the topic and issue covered. The publication is sold with the idea that the publisher is not required to render accounting, officially permitted, or otherwise, qualified services. If advice is necessary, legal, or professional, a practiced individual in the profession should be ordered.

From a Declaration of Principles, which was accepted and approved by a committee of the American Bar Association and a committee of publishers and associations.

In no way is it legal to reproduce, duplicate, or transmit any part of this document in either electronic means or printed format. Recording of this publication is strictly prohibited, and any storage of this document is not allowed unless with written permission from the publisher. All rights reserved.

The information provided herein is stated to be truthful and consistent, in that any liability, in terms of inattention or otherwise, by any usage or abuse of any policies, processes, or directions contained within is the solitary and utter responsibility of the recipient reader. Under no circumstances will any legal responsibility or blame be held against the publisher for any reparation, damages, or monetary loss due to the information herein, either directly or indirectly.

Respective authors own all copyrights not held by the publisher.

The information herein is offered for informational purposes solely. The presentation of the information is without contract or any type of guarantee assurance.

The trademarks that are used are without any consent, and the publication of the trademark is without permission or backing by the trademark owner. All trademarks and brands within this book are for clarifying purposes only and are owned by the owners themselves, not affiliated with this document.

Dedication

To our parents, who provided us with an outstanding education and an awesome outlook on life!

To our five children and four grandchildren, who inspire us to teach them to think outside the box and to NEVER give up!

To each other, exemplifying the depths of love and compassion as well as rekindling the entrepreneurial spirit.

Acknowledgements

THIS BOOK IS part of a journey.

The people we want to thank who have nurtured us along this path include former staff at REI. They believed in Sally, and we are grateful. Our friends who stuck with Sally through an illness that we thought would never quit. Well, it did, and we are making up for lost time.

Our mentors, Buck Rizvi of Health Profits Academy, Jeff Walker of Product Launch Academy, Dr. Steven Sisskind of Real Dose Nutrition, Russell Brunson of DotComSecrets Ignite, Jon Benson of Sellerator, Valerie Hylen of One Source Coaching, and Victoria LaBalme of Rock The Room, you all have sparked a different part of creativity in us.

Our spiritual guides: oh, you are many. Particular thanks to Abraham, Wayne Dyer, Eckhardt Tolle, Oprah Winfrey, Deepak Chopra, Louise Hay, and Maya Angelou. You inspire and change lives—at least one person at a time and in very big ways.

Our friends in this health journey: Luis Rojas, Rachel Behl, and Donna Gates, —thank you for your encouragement and your teachings along the way.

Health practitioners Dr. Sang Lee, Lucy Postolov, Lee Pulos, and Dr. Sunny Lee. - Wow, you guys are awesome.

Dr. Dewayne Smith in Panama. Yes, you too, are a Wow.

Dr. Raphael Mechoulam—thank you for your keen eye and inquisitive mind, as well as your perseverance in the field of endocannabinoid science.

You are all awesome. And we are grateful.

Disclaimer
Health and Safety Warning

The authors of this book are not dispensing medical advice or prescribing the use of this or any technique as a form of treatment for physical, emotional, or medical problems. The information in this book is not a substitute for medical care and advice by your personal physician, directly or indirectly.

The intent of these authors is only to offer information of a general nature to help you in your quest for emotional, mental, and physical well-being. In the event that you use any of the information in this book for yourself or your loved ones, which is your constitutional right, the author and the publisher assume no responsibility for your actions.

The ideas and facts in this document are not intended as substitutes for proper medical advice. Always consult your physician or health care professional before embarking on any new protocol or taking any new supplement—particularly if you are pregnant, nursing, or elderly or if you have a chronic or recurring condition. Any application of the ideas in this document is at the reader's sole discretion and risk.

The authors of this document make no warranty of any nature in regard to the content of this document including, but not limited to, any implied warranties for any particular purpose. The authors are not liable or responsible to any person or entity for any errors contained in this

Sally Schutz, M.D. & Bayne Boyes, FCPA

document or for any special, incidental, or consequential damage caused or allegedly caused directly or indirectly by the information within.

Screenshots in this book are from publicly accessible field archives. All images are copyrights of their respective owners. None of the owners have sponsored or endorsed this publication. Every effort has been made to verify and to acknowledge information and resources of information provided. The authors assume no responsibility or liability in any way for errors, omissions, or contrary interpretation on the subject matter within. Any perceived errors of people or organizations are unintentional. The reader of this publication assumes responsibility for the use of this information. No guarantees of well-being are made. The authors reserve the right to make alterations and assumes no responsibility or liability whatsoever on behalf of any reader of this information.

About the Authors

SALLY SCHUTZ, M.D., retired ophthalmic surgeon, lecturer, teacher, and life coach for Flourishing Fully, recovered from a devastating illness, chronic Lyme disease in 2015. Her recovery was indeed a miracle and changed her life forever with a profound connection to the Universe. She has pursued her passion of serving the Universe by coaching her students in bulletproofing their health, guiding people with chronic illness to regain their health, and teaching tools to align their energy with Universal Laws of Abundance and Connection. She is dedicated to helping people bulletproof their energy, mitochondria and endocannabinoid system.

Dr. Sally, as she has been called by her patients for decades, envisions her soul's purpose as creating bulletproof mindfulness for her clients, as well as raising the consciousness of the planet to a frequency of love, joy, and well-being.

Bayne Boyes FCPA, FCMA feels that his calling in life has been to help others. Professionally he helped organizations (individuals; nonprofits and small businesses) to 'right the ship.' For years, he was the CEO of HANS, Health Action Network Society, a nonprofit health education society in Vancouver. HANS gathered research and established a substantial library in the alternative health area that was effective in helping many people revitalize their health. This society organized events and attracted leading health scientists in North America and Europe.

Sally Schutz, M.D. & Bayne Boyes, FCPA

Bayne has been researching health issues for 20 years and has himself a substantial health library. He is passionate about this opportunity to help people regain and achieve optimal health. Energetically, he pursues his passions with Sally as a partner in Flourish Fully Nutrients, L.P, and in Flourishing Fully, a website dedicated to helping people achieve maximal health with innovative quantum energy information, classes and coaching.

Table of Contents

	Acknowledgements · vii	
	Disclaimer Health and Safety Warning · · · · · · · · · · · · · · · ·ix	
	About the Authors ·xi	
	Introduction· xvii	
Chapter 1	The History of Chinese Medicine · · · · · · · · · · · · · · · · · · 1	
	Chinese Medicine—Written History· · · · · · · · · · · · · · · · 1	
	Traditional Chinese Medicine and Cannabis· · · · · · · · · 4	
	Acupuncture and Cannabis· 6	
Chapter 2	The History of Indian Medicine· 8	
	A Brief Insight into Ayurveda · 8	
	Traditional Indian Medicine and Cannabis · · · · · · · · · · 9	
Chapter 3	Marijuana vs. Cannabinoid Oil from Hemp— What's the Difference? · 13	
	Differences Between Marijuana and Hemp · · · · · · · · · 13	
	Marijuana vs. Hemp Oils · 18	
Chapter 4	Healing History of Marijuana· 20	
	Ancient Egypt · 20	
	Ancient Greece · 22	
	Islamic World and Marijuana · 22	
	Modern Ages · 23	
	Marijuana as a Medicine: A Timeline· · · · · · · · · · · · · · 24	
Chapter 5	Healing History of Hemp Oils · 29	
	Traditional Chinese Medicine · 29	
	Traditional Indian Medicine· 30	

	What Makes Hemp Oil So Special?	31
	Hemp and Hemp Oil Throughout History: A Timeline	32
Chapter 6	Health Benefits of Marijuana and Hemp Success Stories	36
	Story 1: Marijuana stops child's severe seizures	*36*
	Story 2: Marijuana helps one woman overcome cachexia	39
	Story 3: Marijuana reduces essential tremor symptoms and tremor associated with Parkinson's disease	*40*
	Story 4: Marijuana reduces vomiting and nausea in complicated pregnancy	41
	Story 5: Woman beats lung cancer with cannabis oil	41
	Story 6: Marijuana cures insomnia	43
	Story 7: ALS patient benefits from smoking cannabis	43
	Summary	44
Chapter 7	Cannabinoid Patent	46
	Marijuana Patent Belongs to…	47
Chapter 8	Discovery of the Endocannabinoid System by Dr. R. Mechoulam	49
	Who is Dr. Raphael Mechoulam?	49
	What is the Endocannabinoid System?	50
	What is the Purpose of the Endocannabinoid System?	52
	The Endocannabinoid System and Bones	54
	The Endocannabinoid System and Inflammation of the Joints	54
	The Endocannabinoid System and the Brain	55
	The Endocannabinoid System and Immunity	58

	The Endocannabinoid System and Inflammation in the Body · · · · · · · · · · · · · · · · · · · 59
	The Endocannabinoid System and Cardiovascular Benefits · 60
	Endocannabinoid System and Diabetes · · · · · · · · · · · 61
	The Endocannabinoid System and Phantom Limb Pain · 62
	The Endocannabinoid System and PTSD · · · · · · · · · · 62
	The Endocannabinoid System and Anxiety · · · · · · · · · 62
	The Endocannabinoid System and Neural Pain · · · · · 63
	The Endocannabinoid System and Migraines · · · · · · · 63
	The Endocannabinoid System and Chronic Vomiting Disorder · 64
	The Endocannabinoid System and Fibromyalgia · 64
	The Endocannabinoid System and Multiple Sclerosis · 64
	The Endocannabinoid System and ALS · · · · · · · · · · · · 65
	The Endocannabinoid System and AIDS · · · · · · · · · · · 65
	The Endocannabinoid System and Cancer · · · · · · · · · 65
	Other Possibilities that Involve the Endocannabinoid System · 66
	What's next for Endocannabinoid Science? · · · · · · · · 66
Chapter 9	What is The Entourage Effect? · · · · · · · · · · · · · · · · · · 69
	What Does It Really Mean? · 69
	What are Terpenes? · 70
	What are Sterols? · 72
Chapter 10	Mitochondrial Disease · 74
	mTOR Pathways · 76
	CBD and the mTOR pathway · · · · · · · · · · · · · · · · · · · 77
Chapter 11	CBD Oil · 79
	CBD Oil—Basics · 79
	CBG—Cannabigerol · 80

CBD Oil is Not Psychoactive · 81
The Legal Status of CBD Oil · 81
Chapter 12 Why Are Cannabinoids Better than Prescription
Drugs for Pain, Anxiety, and Sleep? · · · · · · · · · · · · · · · · · 82
Conclusion · 89

Introduction

THANK YOU FOR purchasing our book, *The Anti-Aging Miracle of Hemp-Derived CBD Oil: 5,000 Years of Healing the Body and the Mind.*

The cannabis plant itself has been used for medical purposes since ancient times. Medical cannabis was an essential tool for treating numerous diseases and illnesses. Furthermore, the plant also had important roles in other aspects of life, and its importance was documented by numerous scholars. This book will take you on a fascinating journey back to ancient times, where you'll get to see how medical cannabis is deeply connected with ancient Indian and Chinese medicine.

Then, we'll take a giant leap to the modern ages and discuss the role of medical cannabis today, its benefits for the endocannabinoid system (ECS), and the numerous studies that prove the beneficial effects of this plant. Furthermore, the book will inform and inspire you about all aspects of using medical cannabis, the success stories of people who've used it, and what we can expect in the near future.

And don't worry, the book won't bombard you with a bunch of technical or medical terms that most people don't know, understand and don't care about.

Promise!

Sally Schutz, M.D. & Bayne Boyes, FCPA

The primary aim of this book is to educate people about the ECS, what its purpose is, and how medical cannabis can be used as a natural remedy to bring balance to a person's system. The book is fact-based and is an excellent resource for information about the endocannabinoid system and medical cannabis.

This book also provides an abundance of fun facts, interesting stories, photos, useful info, and much more. No need to wait. Start reading today.

Thank you for participating in the evolution of a major new shift in healthcare.

CHAPTER 1

The History of Chinese Medicine

TRADITIONAL CHINESE MEDICINE refers to an ancient practice that is still used by millions of people around the world, even in the era of modern scientific medicine. The essential part of Chinese medicine is the belief that the *microcosm*, or the *individual*, is the integral part of the *macrocosm*, or *forces of nature*.

Traditional Chinese medicine includes a wide range of medical practices that were developed thousands of years ago. These practices include the well-known herbal medicine regimen, massage or *Tui na*, acupuncture, exercise or *qigong*, dietary therapies, etc.

Chinese Medicine—Written History

The first existing records of medical practices can be traced to the first people or tribes that lived in a particular area. In ancient times, people were hunters and gatherers. They ate the meat of the animals they caught and the produce they gathered. Injuries, diseases, and other illnesses were extremely frequent, and people (usually women) found practical ways to help relieve pain or cure some illness. Most herbal remedies that we use today have their origins in traditional medicine.

However, the written history of Chinese traditional medicine has evolved over the last 3,000 years. Archaeological findings from the famous

Sally Schutz, M.D. & Bayne Boyes, FCPA

Shang[1] dynasty revealed various medical writings that were imprinted on divination bones. Early *shamans* (most of them women) used scapula bones to perform divination rituals. Later, these bones were used for writing.

Archaeologists also found stone and bone needles, which led Joseph Needham[2] to assume that acupuncture, which is still widely popular today, had been carried out during the years of the Shang dynasty.

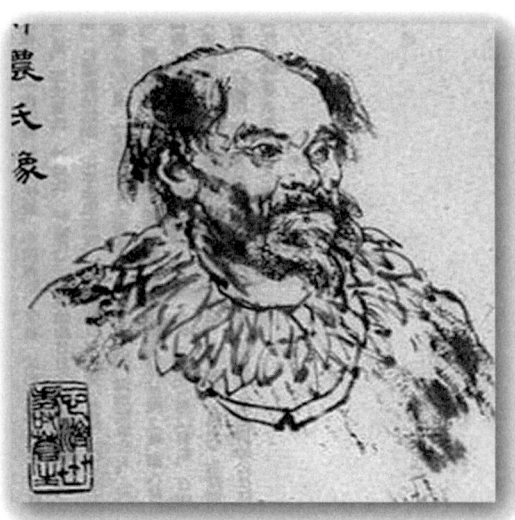

Shennong
(photo courtesy of <u>wikipedia.org</u>)

In 1973, archaeologists discovered eleven texts about medicine. They were written on silk. These texts provided a detailed insight into sophisticated medical techniques practiced in the early period of Chinese history. They discussed the importance of exercise, a healthy diet, and herbal therapy.

Chinese medicine relied on herbs and plants to cure various diseases and establish a balance in one's body. An extensive text, *Wu Shi ER Bing Fang* (*Prescriptions for Fifty-Two Ailments*), described the beneficial effects of herbs and plants.

---

1 Dates given for founding of Shang dynasty vary from 1760 to 1520 BC, as well as dates for the dynasty's fall, which happened between 1122 and 1030 BC.
2 Joseph Needham was a British scientist, sociologist, and historian known for his scientific research on the history of Chinese science.

The Anti-Aging Miracles of Hemp-Derived CBD Oil

When talking about herbs in Chinese medicine, it's important to mention Shennong.[3] According to many legends, he tasted more than 100 herbs a day to assess their quality and determine if they could be used as cures for various ailments. Shennong is said to have been poisoned on numerous occasions in the course of his experiments. There's also a book that's attributed to Shennong, *Classic of the Agriculture Emperor's Materia Medica*. The book mentions 365 remedies or medicines (consisting of 252 plants, sixty-seven animals, and forty-six minerals).

The editor of today's *Materia Medica*, Tao Hong-Jing, classifies herbs into three categories:

- upper-class herbs—nontoxic tonics that nourish and strengthen the body
- middle-grade herbs—tonics that possess therapeutic qualities
- lower-grade herbs—herbs that treat ailments and diseases or possess certain levels of toxicity

This classification system is important because it gives us a brief insight into the core of traditional Chinese medicine. The primary principle of Chinese medicine was that it's better to strengthen the body and prevent illness than to fight illness when it has already taken over the body. Back then, not taking care of your health and waiting for a disease to manifest before doing anything about it was considered foolish.

By the year 400 AD, all principles and doctrines of traditional Chinese medicine were in writing. The most important work from the period

---
3 Shennong, or Emperor of the Five Grains, was an emperor of China and a cultural hero. He has been given credit for inventing the hoe, the plowshare, and the plow.

between 300 BC and 400 AD is *The Yellow Emperor's Inner Classic*, which historians regard as the most unique compilation of all medical knowledge from that time.

Traditional Chinese Medicine and Cannabis

As seen above, traditional Chinese medicine relied on the use of different herbs and plants to protect one's body and keep it healthy. Most herbs that were integral parts of traditional Chinese medicine are still used today (e.g. ginger or Ginkgo biloba). However, what most people don't know is that cannabis also played an important role in medical practices throughout the history of China.

For example, we already know what acupuncture is; you likely have already tried it or you know someone who has. But did you know that acupuncture and cannabis are connected? According to a number of studies, acupuncture is beneficial for the endocannabinoid system, just like cannabis.

This plant has a long history in traditional Chinese medicine; it's one of the fifty fundamental and most important herbs of Chinese medicine and was praised for its ability to treat various symptoms and different diseases.

The first person who mentioned and documented benefits of cannabis was none other than Shennong. In his book, mentioned above, Shennong mentioned hemp elixir, which was most likely a tea of flowers and leaves. Furthermore, Shennong received hemp as a payment on numerous occasions.

The Divine Farmer's *Materia Medica*, which is also regarded as the oldest pharmacopoeia,[4] reveals that cannabis is a powerful plant that can

---

[4] Official publication containing a list of medicinal drugs with effects and usage directions. In past, the term referred to an herbal reference book.

The Anti-Aging Miracles of Hemp-Derived CBD Oil

prevent and treat more than 100 different ailments, like gout, malaria, rheumatism, absentmindedness, etc. It describes the seeds as boosting the qi and helping to avoid senility.

A few centuries after Shennong described all the powerful benefits of cannabis, a Chinese medical text suggested that cannabis could treat bacterial infections, vomiting, and hemorrhages.

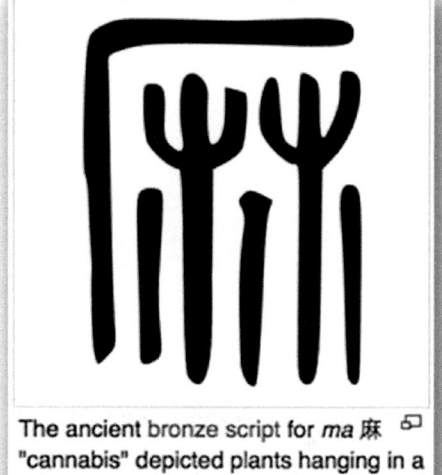

The ancient bronze script for *ma* 麻 "cannabis" depicted plants hanging in a shed.

Shennong wasn't the only one who experimented with plants to discover all their benefits. An ancient Chinese physician, Hua Tuo (140–208 AD), was the first person to use cannabis as an anesthetic (*Book of the Later Han*). Even the term for anesthesia that is used in China today is composed of the Chinese characters for hemp and intoxication.

So, how did he do it? Hua Tuo came up with the idea to dry the plant and turn it into powder. Then, he would mix it with wine for external and internal administration. The physician performed surgeries in which he removed affected tissues with systemic and local administration of cannabis-enriched wine as a powerful anesthetic. Furthermore, Hua Tuo also used an acupuncture technique whose primary purpose was to control the pain.

The connection between acupuncture and cannabis is quite interesting. Let's take a closer look.

Acupuncture and Cannabis

Acupuncture is a type of alternative medicine and an essential part of traditional Chinese medicine. It involves thin needles that are inserted into one's body at acupuncture points. The practice is still widely popular and is known for its ability to provide general relaxation, as well as relief from chronic pain, back pain, etc. However, the mechanisms underlying its beneficial effects are still largely unknown.

Inserting needles into acupuncture points aims to influence the flow—or *qi*, the vital energy of the body. Chinese physicians believe that lack of movement and stagnation of this energy causes dysfunction and pain in the organism.

In many cases, acupuncture is coupled with *moxibustion*, which is the process in which the herb mugwort is burned close to the person's skin or in a rolled cigarette as a concentrated and unique source of heat.

What's this got to do with cannabis? The answer is: everything.

Many scholars who spent their lives reading and analyzing texts concerning traditional Chinese medicine discovered that the herb used by Chinese medical practitioners wasn't mugwort but rather was *cannabis*.

In fact, mugwort was only used as the wrap for the cigarette, while cannabis was the "filling" inside. Chinese physicians were smoking out the patients because the smoke stimulated the skin with heat. Additionally, it was believed that the smoke *of cigar* had healing properties. (http://www.thenorthwestleaf.com/-pages/articles/post/traditional-chinese-medicine-how-marijuana-has-been-used-for-centuries).

The medical practitioners would first smoke out the patients and then use needles to stimulate the movement of ch*i*.

Moxibustion and acupuncture were highly popular in China. In fact, they were considered as an essential part of a systematic approach to health.

CHAPTER 2

The History of Indian Medicine

TRADITIONAL MEDICINE OF India features the practices of combining religion and science. A wide range of medical approaches has their roots in religious texts. Here, we're going to discuss the most notable one—Ayurveda.

A Brief Insight into Ayurveda

Traditional Indian medicine revolves around Ayurveda. It is a 5,000-year-old system of natural healing that has its origin in the *Vedic* culture. Ayurvedic practices and healing methods are still used today as part of alternative medicine.

The earliest Sanskrit works on Ayurveda suggest that medical science, in general, is divided into eight components. They are:

- medicine of the body or general medicine
- pediatrics or treatment of children
- extraction of foreign objects from the body and surgical methods
- treatment of diseases that affect eyes, nose, ears, mouth, etc.
- pacification of people whose minds are affected by possessive spirits
- toxicology
- rejuvenation and usage of tonics to increase strength, lifespan, and intellect
- treatments for increasing sexual pleasure, viability and volume of semen, and aphrodisiacs

Physicians who practiced Ayurveda regarded physical existence, personality, and mental existence as one unique unit. Each of these three elements has the ability to affect the others. Here, we can draw a parallel between the traditional medicines of China and India. Both promoted healthy lifestyles and suggested that in order to stay healthy, people needed to have the balance between mind, body, and soul or spirit. Instead of prescribing treatment for some diseases when an individual felt sick, both types of medicine promoted the idea of a vital balance to prevent various ailments.

According to Ayurveda, physical pain can also influence the mental abilities of a person, making them feel stressed out, a condition that automatically affects a person's character and personality.

In order to establish this recommended equilibrium, Ayurvedic practitioners used herbs and plants as a part of natural healing.

Besides Ayurveda, traditional Indian medicine also included a number of other practices, most of which don't exist today. However, Ayurveda and some other native medical traditions managed to stay alive and are currently in use.

These healing traditions in India continued to exist even after Muslims introduced their healing methods in 11th century.

In the 18th century, when British monarchs conquered India, Western medicine was introduced. During this time, the usage of Ayurveda practices declined to some degree, only to be embraced anew after India gained independence in 1947.

Traditional Indian Medicine and Cannabis

Cannabis was important for religious ceremonies in India as well as medicinal purposes. For many centuries of country's rich history, the people of India have used cannabis in many different forms. The earliest mention of cannabis in India can be found in the *Vedas*, which were compiled between 2000 and

1400 BC. According to the *Vedas*, cannabis is one of five sacred plants. The texts also suggested that guardian angels live in cannabis leaves.

The *Vedas* also state that cannabis is the source of happiness and helps people retain their happiness and let go of all their fears. These scripts also mention that cannabis relieves stress and anxiety.

Ancient Indian texts reveal that physicians recognized the psychoactive properties of cannabis and used the plant to treat various ailments and diseases. For example:

- insomnia
- headache
- gastrointestinal diseases
- pain (even pain during childbirth)

Cannabis has played an important role in Ayurvedic medicine. The plant was even included into *Homeopathic Pharmacopoeia of India* in 1971. Some of the benefits of cannabis mentioned in the pharmacopoeia are:

- Leaves are beneficial for "deterging" the brain.
- Cannabis juice removes dandruff when applied onto the scalp.
- Cannabis juice relieves earache when dropped into the ear.
- Powdered leaves speed up granulation when applied to fresh wounds.
- Cannabis has sedative properties.
- Cannabis helps with hemorrhoids.
- Cannabis demonstrates pain-relieving properties.
- Cannabis relieves pain associated with migraines.
- Cannabis helps bronchodilation with asthma.
- Cannabis is an effective remedy for dysentery.
- Cannabis oil helps with rheumatic pain.

The Anti-Aging Miracles of Hemp-Derived CBD Oil

However, after being pressured by the United States, which banned the usage of cannabis (even for medical purposes), India enacted a law in 1985 forbidding the use of this plant. In some parts of the country, though, Ayurvedic practitioners still use cannabis as part of their treatments, and students throughout India still learn about the powerful benefits of this plant.

90   HOMOEOPATHIC PHARMACOPOEA OF INDIA

CANNABIS INDICA

(Can. Ind.)

Bot. Name	: Cannabis sative Lica	Family: Cannabinaceae
Synonym	: Cannabis indica Lamk.	
Description	: Strong smelling, stout, erect annual herb, branched or nearly simple, 1-3.5 meters in height. Leaves alternate, thin, long petioled; the blade digitate with 3-7 long lanceolate or linear-lanceolate, long acuminate leaflets.	
Microscopical	: Leaves and bracts dorsiventral. Upper epidermis bears unicellular, pointed, conical curred trichomes with enlarged bases containing cystoliths of calcium carbonate. Mesophyll contains cluster crystals of calcium oxalate in many cells and consists of usually one layer of palisade cells and spongy tissue. Trichomes on the lower epidermis conical, longer but without cystoliths. Numerous glandular trichomes, senile or with a multicellular stalk and secreting head of about eight radiating clubshaped cells, secreting cleorisin; present in the lower epidermis especially on mid-rib.	
Habitat	: Considered a native of Western Central Asia but practically naturalized in the sub-Himalayan tract in India and is abundantly nxt with waste lands from Puajab eastwards to Bengal and Bibar and extending southwards to Deccan cultivated.	
History and Authority	: Introduced into Homoeopathic practice in 1841 by Dr. Trinks, Atig. Hom. Zeir. XX 268. Allen's Encyclop. Mat. Med. Vol 11. 448; X 409.	
Part Used	: Leaves.	
Preparation	: (a) Mother Tincture	Drug strength 1/10

Cannabis indica, moist magma containing solids 100 g and plant moisture approximately 180 ml 280 g

Strong Alcohol 850 ml

To make one thousand millilitres of the Mother Tincture.

(b) Potencies:

2x with Strong Alcohol. 3x and higher with dispersing alcohol

Figure 1 Cannabis in the Official Pharmacopoeia of India (courtesy of antiquecannabisbook.com)

CANNABIS SATIVA

(Can. Sat.)

Bot. Name	: Cannabis sativa Linn. Family: Cannabinaceae
Synonyms	: English: Hemp, Gallow grass; French: Chanvic; German: Flanf.
Description	: Strong, smelling, stout, erect annual herb, branched or nearly simple, 1-3.5 metres. Leaves alternate, thin, long petioled; the blade digitate with 3-7 long lanceolate or liner-lanceolate, large toothed, long acuminate leaflets.
Macroscopal	: Flattened, cylindrical, rough dull dusky green masses consisting of the branched upper part of the stem, bearing braces, bracteoles, pistillate flowers or fruits matted together by resinous secretion. Stem thin, straight, cylindrical, longitudinally furrowed; bracts 1.5 to 2 cm long. Simple or lobed with 2 small substate stipulate stipales; bracteoles in pairs in the axil of bract, boat-shaped with acute apices, incurved at the base to enclose the flower or fruit, flowers formed in the axil of each bracteole and each consists of an ovary enclosed by hairy membraneous perianth; ovary 2mm long, surmounted by 2 long brownish red hairy stigmas. Fruits achenes, few, 5-6 mm long, 4mm wide, ovoid, glossy green or yellowish green, single seeded.
Microscopical	: Leaves and bract dorsiventral. Upper epidermis bears unicellular, pointed, conical, curved trichomes with enlarged base containing cystoliths of calcium carbonate. Mesophyll contains cluster crystals of calcium oxalate in many cells and consists of usually one layer of palisade cells and spongy tissue. Trichomes on the lower epidermis conical, longer but without cytoliths. Numerous glandular trichomes, sessile or with a multicellular stalk and a secreting head of about eight radiating club-shaped cells, secreting oleo-resin present in the lower epidermis especially on mid-rib. Bracteoles have undifferentiated mesophyll and bear on lower surface numerous glandular trichomes. Stem has well developed bundles or pericyclic fibres; phloem contains large unbranched laticiferous tubes; cluster crystals of calcium oxalate present in both cortex and pith.
Habitat	: Considered a native of Western Central Asia but practically naturalized in the sub-Himalayan tract in India and is abundantly met/cultivated from Punjab eastwards to Bengal and Bihar and extending southwards to Deccan.
History and Authority	: Allen's Encyclop. Mat. Med. Vol. II. 492
Part Used	: Flowering tops of both male and female.
Preparation	: (a) Mother Tincture Drug Strength 1/10

Cannabis Sativa moist magma containing solids 100 g and plant moisture 200 ml............300 g

Purified Water..100 ml

Strong Alcohol..730 ml

To make one thousand millilitres of the Mother Tincture.

(b) Potencies:

2x to contain one part Mother Tincture, two parts Purified Water, seven parts Strong Alcohol. 3x and higher with dispensing alcohol.

Old Method	: Class III, Class I, page 258, 257.

Figure 2 Cannabis in the Official Pharmacopoeia of India (courtesy of antiquecannabisbook.com)

CHAPTER 3

Marijuana vs. Cannabinoid Oil from Hemp—What's the Difference?

BEFORE WE LEARN the difference between oils from marijuana and hemp, we have to know the difference between the plants themselves. Most people assume marijuana and hemp are just synonyms for one term, but that's not quite true. The general information available regarding the plants is limited, and the data found on various websites prove to be inaccurate.

Therefore, before we start discussing all the benefits of medical marijuana, or even hemp oils, we simply must know how they differ. Let's find out.

Differences Between Marijuana and Hemp

GENETICS
Both marijuana and hemp belong to the cannabis family. We've already seen the immense importance of cannabis for ancient cultures, societies, and their medical practices. In fact, scientists and historians believe that cannabis poses as one of the oldest domesticated crops.

Sally Schutz, M.D. & Bayne Boyes, FCPA

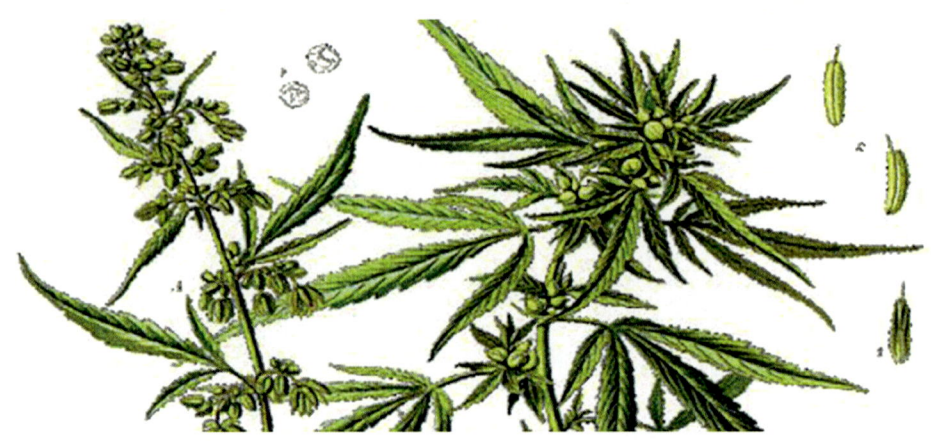

Cannabis Sativa

Illustration from Kohler's book of medicinal plants from 1897

Cannabis is characterized by a tall and sturdy plant structure. It was grown by early civilizations for use in textiles, oils, fabrics, ropes, etc. These cannabis plants were bred with other types of plants with similar characteristics. These practices created a new type of cannabis that we call "hemp."

People discovered that some cannabis plants had psychoactive properties and they were primarily used for medicinal purposes. We know these plants today by the name "marijuana."

The most notable differences between marijuana and hemp manifest themselves in the cultivation methods and the genetic parentage.

There are two main types of cannabis:

- *Cannabis Indica*
- *Cannabis Sativa*

Both marijuana and hemp belong to the Cannabis Sativa family.

The Anti-Aging Miracles of Hemp-Derived CBD Oil

THC Content

Tetrahydrocannabinol, or THC, is the chemical that is responsible for the psychoactive effects of marijuana.

Cannabis plants contain some 480 natural components, of which 111 are different *cannabinoids*. The more well-known are:

- Cannabigerols (CBG)
- Cannabichromenes (CBC)
- Cannabidiols (CBD)
- Tetrahydrocannabinols (THC)
- Cannabinol (CBN) and Cannabinodiol (CBDL)
- Cannabicyclol (CBL)
- Cannabielsoin (CBE)
- Cannabitriol (CBT)

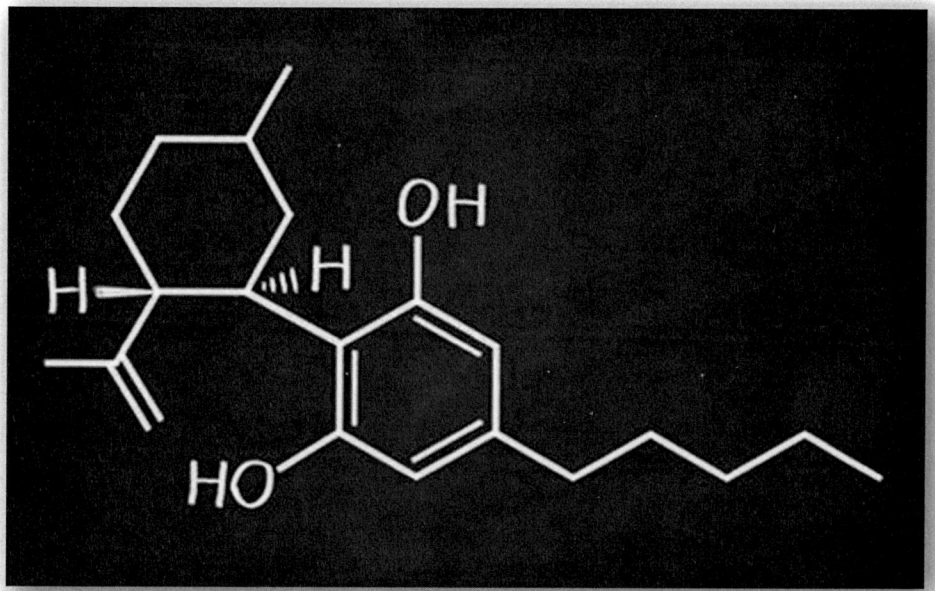

Image courtesy of Raimundo79: shutterstock.com

While THC is the most famous, CBD is probably the most abundant cannabinoid, contributing up to 40 percent of cannabis resin.

• • •

THC was first discovered and isolated in the early 1960s by Israeli scientist, Dr. Raphael Mechoulam. At this time, Dr. Mechoulam was a postdoctoral student when he noticed that, even though active compounds from cocaine or morphine were isolated, nobody had conducted such a process with marijuana.

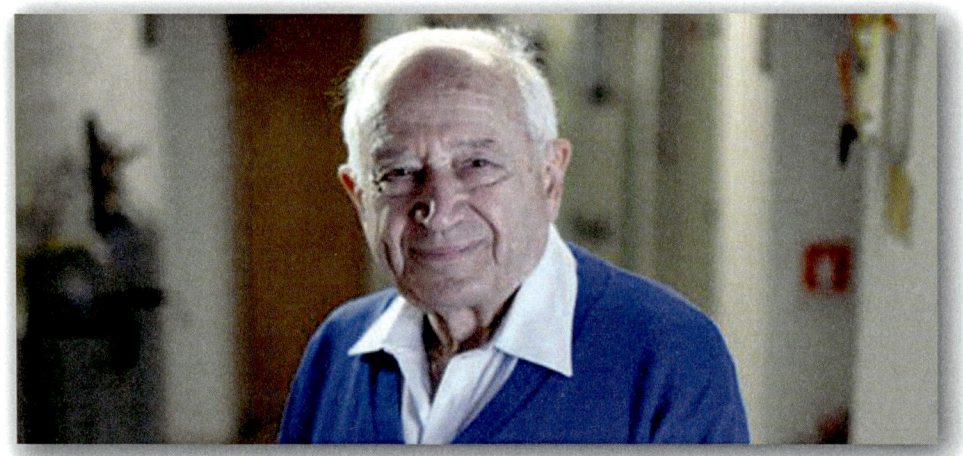

Dr. Raphael Mechoulam (courtesy of www.israel21c.org)

Dr. Mechoulam's motivation was so strong that he even broke the law trying to obtain marijuana from his friends at the police department. Luckily, the famous scientist succeeded in isolating THC in 1964. This revelation marked the start of a prolific career dedicated to cannabis research (more on Dr. Mechoulam further in the book).

Hemp contains low levels of THC. Many countries have established a maximum level of THC for various products; Canada was the first to establish a limit 0.3% which became the standard in the rest of the world too. Everything above that limit is defined as marijuana.

As mentioned above, THC is the chemical that is the primary "culprit" for the "high" or "stoned" effects of marijuana. Medical marijuana's THC content is between 5% and 20%. Furthermore, prize marijuana strains can contain from 25% to 30% of THC.

THC content is one of the most important differences between marijuana and hemp. Another chemical compound found in cannabis plants is *cannabidiol* (CBD). According to some studies, CBD reduces the effects of THC.

Hemp plants contain higher levels of CBD and lower levels of THC. On the other hand, marijuana plants contain higher levels of THC and lower amounts of CBD.

CULTIVATION

Considering the fact that marijuana and hemp are grown for different uses, their cultivation conditions are also different. In order to make sure marijuana plants develop maximum levels of THC, cultivators need to provide a level of attention that is somewhat close to grow-room conditions. On the other hand, hemp doesn't need that much attention. It is usually grown outdoors to maximize its size. Unlike marijuana, hemp plants grow faster and taller.

PRODUCTION AND LEGAL STATUS

Production of all cannabis plants is strictly illegal in the United States. However, other countries don't have such harsh rules. For example, hemp is grown in more than thirty countries. Top hemp-producing countries include China, Chile, and the European Union. Cultivation of hemp in Canada is also increasing.

However, although production and cultivation of hemp is as illegal as cultivation and production of marijuana, the United States *allows* the importation of hemp products. The Hemp Industry Association reveals that $500 million worth of hemp products are imported into the US each year. Nowadays, many body care products such as foot creams, hand creams, and lotions are made out of hemp.

Marijuana vs. Hemp Oils

The primary differences between marijuana and hemp oils are in the content and usage. While hemp plants are primarily male and lack budding flowers, marijuana plants are female, which plays an important role in making oils as well.

Hemp oils have a strict limit of up to 0.3% THC content making them NON-psychoactive, while marijuana (as well as marijuana oils) has significantly higher levels of this compound.

Marijuana is primarily used for recreational purposes, although the medicinal benefits are surfacing at a rapid pace in recent years; some researches even state it can slow down the spread of cancerous cells.

Other uses of marijuana include:

- glaucoma
- dandruff
- obesity
- asthma
- multiple sclerosis
- pain
- hemorrhoids
- leprosy

The Anti-Aging Miracles of Hemp-Derived CBD Oil

- urinary infections
- prevention of organ rejection after kidney transplant[5]

Hemp oils or hemp-derived CBD oils are also used for healing purposes. They can also be used for:

- cooking (it's rich in nutrients)
- moisturizing after showers
- production of paints
- bio-diesel fuel like vegetable oils
- production of foods, lotions, soaps, etc.

Hemp oils are legal and can be obtained without a prescription. They can be freely used around the household since they don't have psychoactive characteristics. In contrast, the legality of marijuana varies from state to state and requires a prescription for its health-related properties.

---

5 A team of scientists from University of South Carolina discovered that THC from marijuana prevents organ rejection after transplants and could be useful for anti-rejection therapy. Findings from this study were published in the *Journal of Leukocyte Biology*.

CHAPTER 4

• • •

Healing History of Marijuana

THE HEALING HISTORY of marijuana can be traced back thousands of years. Chapters one and two already discussed traditional medicine practices of China and India, as well as the importance of cannabis for the treatment of various diseases. However, the Chinese and Indian civilizations weren't the only ones that discovered the amazing benefits of this plant. Let's take a look at the healing history of marijuana in other cultures and societies.

Ancient Egypt

A vast majority of archaeologists agree that marijuana was used for medical purposes in ancient Egypt. This notion contradicts the findings from the early 1930s, when historians and archaeologists never mentioned that marijuana could be an important part of Egypt's medical practices. *What changed?* When deciphering hieroglyphs was finally possible, not all references to medicines and plants found written in ancient papyruses were readable. Only in mid-20th century was the usage of cannabis in ancient Egypt identified and confirmed.

A hieroglyph that referred to marijuana is displayed below.

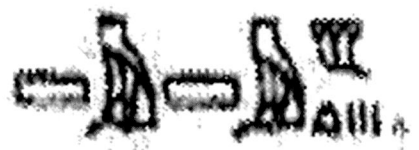

Hieroglyphs are usually read right to left.

The Anti-Aging Miracles of Hemp-Derived CBD Oil

The signs you see on the image above are pronounced as *shm-shm-tu*, and their literal meaning is "the medical marijuana plant."

Medical marijuana is mentioned in these ancient Egyptian texts:

- *The Ramesseum III Papyrus*, 1700 BC
- *Ebers Papyrus*,[6] 1600 BC
- *The Berlin Papyrus*, 1300 BC
- *The Chester Beatty VI Papyrus*, 1300 BC

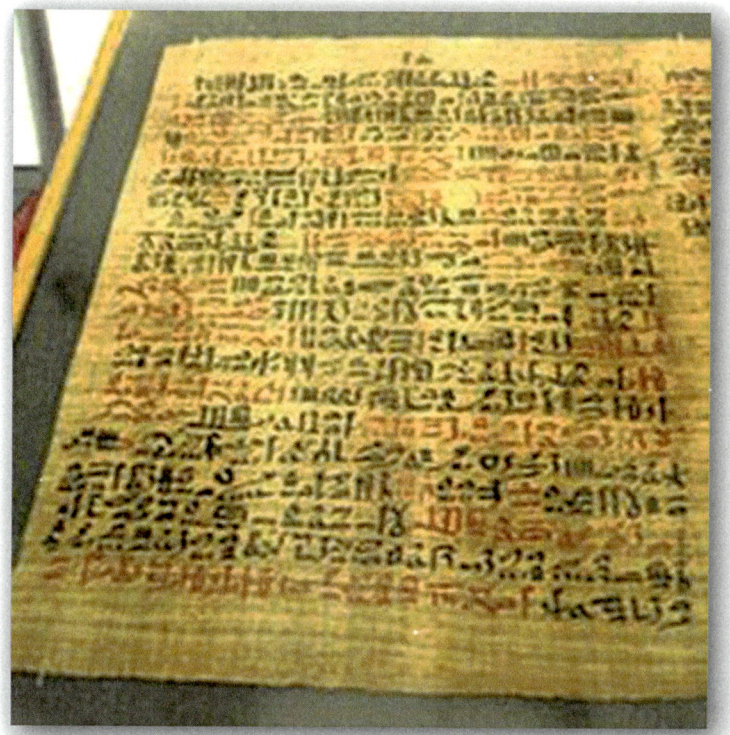

The Ebers Papyrus contains a prescription of medical marijuana for relieving inflammation (courtesy of antiquecannabisbook.com).

---

6 The Ebers Papyrus is unique because, although it's not the oldest recorded mention of cannabis, it is the oldest *complete* textbook regarding medical practices that is still in existence.

Egyptians used marijuana to treat:

- inflammations
- hemorrhoids
- sore eyes

Ancient Greece

Ancient Greeks went one step further than the Egyptians, Indians, and Chinese. They used cannabis for treating both humans and animals. When it comes to animals, they used marijuana to treat sores and wounds on horses.

The most frequent usages of cannabis in humans were for:

- treating nosebleeds
- expelling tapeworms
- treating inflammation
- reducing ear pain

The Greeks came up with a unique way to treat inflammations. They steeped green seeds of cannabis in hot wine or water. After some time, they would take out the seeds and apply the warm extract onto affected areas of the body.

Islamic World and Marijuana

Marijuana was a part of the Islamic world's medical practices in the time frame between the 8th and 18th centuries. In this culture's medicine, marijuana was used for the following properties:

- anti-inflammatory
- antiepileptic

- diuretic
- analgesic
- antipyretic
- anti-emetic properties

Modern Ages

During the mid-19th century, interest in medical marijuana started to increase in Western countries. In that time, several patent medicines used cannabis as a secret ingredient. Before the year 1937, there were more than 2,000 medicines that contained cannabis on the market produced by 280 manufacturers, according to the *Antique Cannabis Book* (antiquecannabisbook.com).

The person who's accredited for introducing the powerful benefits of medical marijuana to the West was William Brooke O'Shaughnessy, an Irish physician. He worked in Calcutta, India as an assistant surgeon and professor of chemistry at the Medical College of Calcutta. Professor O'Shaughnessy conducted a series of experiments with cannabis and used the plant to treat:

- migraines
- muscle spasms
- stomach cramps
- general pain

The popularity of cannabis and its medical benefits kept increasing, which inspired scientists to conduct a number of studies to observe its health effects in humans. For example, in 1964 Dr. Albert Lockhart studied the health effects of marijuana in Jamaica. In his work *Cannabis Unmasked: What is it and Why it Does What it Does*, Dr. Farid F. Youssef writes that

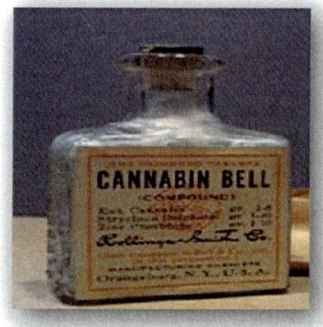

Lockhart discovered that Rastafarians had low glaucoma rates. Together with Manley West, Lockhart developed the pharmaceutical Canasol, which was one of the first cannabis extracts.

Nowadays, the story is quite different. Only a few countries in the world and states in the U.S. allow consumption of marijuana for medical purposes. In general, usage of this plant is strictly forbidden by the law. However, numerous scientists still promote the need to study this plant more thoroughly and use its potential to prevent, treat, and cure a wide range of ailments and diseases.

Marijuana as a Medicine: A Timeline

Now that we've seen how ancient civilizations used marijuana as an integral part of their medicine and studied its impact on modern ages, let's take a look at the timeline of the most important cannabis related events and years from 2900 BC to 2015 AD.

- 2900 BC—Chinese emperor Fu Hsi references marijuana as one of the most popular medicines. This emperor is also praised for bringing civilization to China.
- 2700 BC—Shennong discovers the healing benefits of marijuana.
- 1500 BC—Earliest written reference records the medical properties of marijuana in Chinese pharmacopoeia.
- 1450 BC—The book of Exodus mentions holy anointing oil made of cannabis.
- 1213 BC—Egyptians start using cannabis for inflammations and glaucoma.
- 1000 BC—Indians use a drink of cannabis and milk, called *bhang*, as anesthetic.
- 700 BC—Marijuana is used for treatment of diseases and ailments in the Middle East.
- 600 BC—Indians use marijuana as a cure for leprosy.

The Anti-Aging Miracles of Hemp-Derived CBD Oil

- 200 BC—Ancient Greeks start using marijuana for its healing properties.
- 1 AD—A book attributed to Shennong mentions marijuana as a cure for 100 ailments.
- 30—Jesus uses anointing oil made from cannabis.
- 70—Medical textbooks from ancient Rome suggest that marijuana treats earaches and reduces sexual longing.
- 79—Pliny the Elder mentions medical benefits of cannabis.
- 200—Hua Tuo in China uses cannabis as an anesthetic.
- 800–900—Arabic world uses cannabis as medicine.
- 1500—Muslim doctors start using marijuana to reduce sexuality and sexual desire.
- 1621—Robert Burton, an English clergyman and Oxford scholar, suggests that marijuana is effective in treatment for depression in his book, *The Anatomy of Melancholy*.
- 1840—Queen Victoria uses marijuana to relieve menstrual cramps. In the 1840s, marijuana becomes the mainstream remedy for various ailments in the West.
- 1850—Marijuana is added to the U.S. pharmacopoeia. For almost sixty years, cannabis makes up 50 percent of the medicine sold in the United States.
- 1900—Marijuana is used to treat asthma, loss of appetite, and bronchitis in South Asia.
- 1916—The U.S. Department of Agriculture (USDA) Bulletin 404 predicts mechanized decorticating and harvesting equipment will make hemp America's largest agricultural industry.

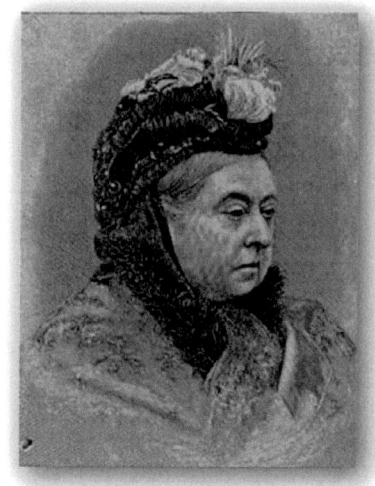

Queen Victoria

- 1918—Pharmaceutical farms in the U.S. grow 60,000 pounds of marijuana annually.
- 1930s—The term *marijuana* becomes popular in the U.S. Pharmaceutical companies start selling marijuana extracts as medicine.
- 1937—President Franklin Roosevelt signs federal legislation prohibiting production, sales and use of cannabis, both hemp and marijuana.
- Aug. 2, 1937—The Marihuana Tax Act of 1937 was passed, placing a tax on the sale of cannabis by dealers. Hemp threatens the interests of paper, cotton, and synthetic fiber industrialists. Harry Anslinger, the first commissioner of the U.S. Treasury Department's Federal Bureau of Narcotics, promotes prohibition and criminalization of drugs including marihuana and hemp. He claims marijuana causes violent behavior.
- 1937—Hemp cultivation declines in the United States.
- 1938—*Reefer Madness* is made, a film demonizing the effects of marijuana
  1939—The AMA is coerced into siding with Anslinger against marijuana.
- 1942—U.S. pharmacopoeia removes marijuana from the list of healing plants.
- 1942—Hemp was greatly needed during WWII as Japan cut off supplies. *Hemp for Victory*, a U.S. war propaganda film, was produced to initiate and stimulate hemp production for the war efforts. Hemp is used in ropes for ships, parachute lines, and fire hoses. Hemp seeds are handed out to farmers.
- 1948—There is a 180-degree turn around during the Cold War, and Anslinger proclaims that marijuana renders its users peaceful and non-violent—an obvious danger to Americans worried about the threat of communism. Other countries participate in this attitude and curtail the growth of hemp and marijuana as well.
- 1970—The Controlled Substances Act categorizes marijuana as a drug with *no accepted medical use*. Marijuana is placed in Schedule

The Anti-Aging Miracles of Hemp-Derived CBD Oil

1. (Drugs in Schedule 1 are classified as possessing immense potential for abuse.) Legal obstacles prohibit marijuana and hemp for medicinal purposes.
- 1976—The Ford Administration and the Drug Enforcement Administration (DEA) prohibit any American research on natural cannabis plants for medicinal purposes. This takes place while the Netherlands actually decriminalizes marijuana.
- 1978—By its Lynn and Erin Compassionate Use Act, New Mexico is among the first states to recognize the healing benefits of marijuana.
- 1988—Allyn Howlett and William Devane use radioimmunoassay techniques to characterize the existence of a cannabinoid receptor in a rat brain.
- 1990—In 1990, Miles Herkenham and fellow researchers announce in the Proceedings of the National Academy of Science that they have mapped the locations of a cannabinoid receptor system in several mammalian species, including man.
- 1992—Dr. Raphael Mechoulam, considered to be the father of the endocannabinoid system, discovers the first endocannabinoid neurotransmitter. He names it *anandamide*. This name is derived from the Sanskrit word for bliss and amide because of the chemical structure of ethanol*amide*.
- November 5, 1996—Proposition 215, the California Compassionate Use Act of 1996, is passed by 55.5 percent of the state's voters, allowing the use of medical cannabis. The act passes in spite of marijuana not having normal FDA testing for safety and efficacy.
- November 3, 1998—Alaska, Oregon, and Washington also legalize medical marijuana. Other states follow suit over the next fifteen years, including Colorado in 2000.
- 2013—A CNN special with Sanjay Gupta airs about marijuana and its health benefits.
- 2014—Maryland, Minnesota, and New York legalize medical marijuana.

- June 22, 2015—Obama's administration and the Department of Health and Human Services remove legal obstacles to marijuana research "effective immediately."
- November 11, 2015—the senate passes legislation that allows Veterans Health Administration doctors to authorize medical marijuana use for patients.

CHAPTER 5

Healing History of Hemp Oils

HEMP OIL HAS a long tradition in medicine, just like another member of Cannabis Sativa family. Furthermore, hemp oil is used in other aspects of life, e.g. skincare and even cooking (as mentioned in chapter three). In this chapter, we're going to discuss the amazing benefits of hemp oils and their long history.

Traditional Chinese Medicine

The first record of using hemp oil as medicine in China go as far back as 4,000 years. Generally, industrial hemp has been used in China for thousands of years and not just as medicine. The hemp was used as food as well as medicine.

According to the ancient texts about traditional Chinese medicine, hemp was used for the purposes listed below:

- anti-inflammation
- antiseptic (preventing growth of bacteria)
- demulcent (soothing and protecting intestinal membrane)
- carrier (the function of carrier oil is to dilute the essential oils, especially in the cases when they have to be applied onto the skin)
- anti-atherosclerotic (hemp oil improves blood flow in the body and regulates blood pressure, which also prevents various cardiovascular diseases)

- diuretic (hemp oil has the amazing ability to improve blood flow through the kidneys and to release excess water)
- edema
- constipation
- tonic for overall health and well-being
- correcting menstrual irregularities and reducing the pain associated with menstrual cramps.

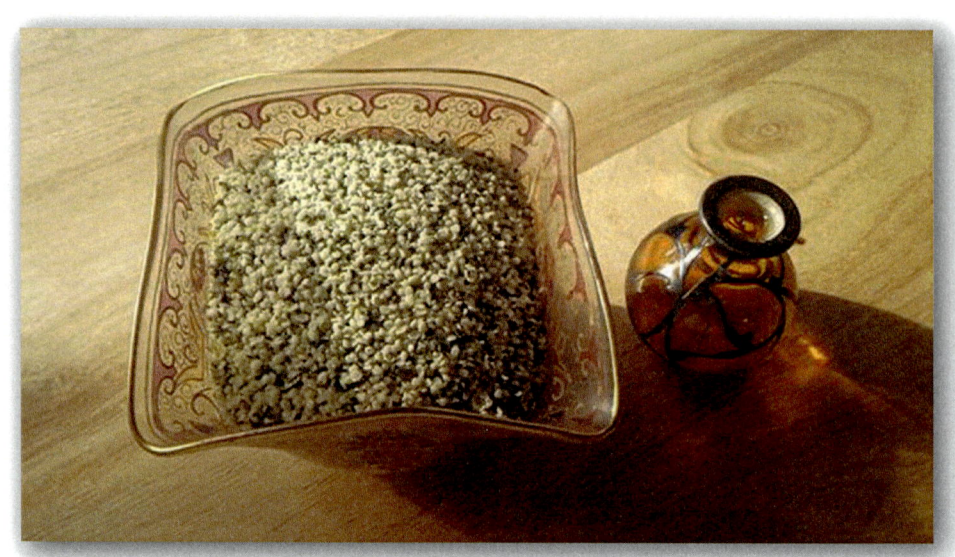

Photo Courtesy of BestCann.Com

Traditional Indian Medicine

Hemp is honored by Indians as one of the "precious things" that were recovered at the birth of the Universe from the primeval sea. According to numerous legends, hemp was taken by Indian gods to gain immortality. Sanskrit texts refer to hemp as *Vijaya*, which means "conquest" because the plant granted victory to all gods who used it.

Hemp oils were used in traditional Indian medicine for its hypnotic, aphrodisiac, and diuretic properties, as well as to treat the following:

- premature ejaculation
- lack of appetite
- headache
- migraine
- insomnia
- indigestion and anorexia
- cough
- gonorrhea
- painful labor

What Makes Hemp Oil So Special?

Throughout history, cultures and civilizations used hemp oil. *So, what makes it so special?* Hemp oil is extracted from the hemp plant. Although all plants of the cannabis family (including marijuana) produce oil, hemp oil is most frequently used. Historians believe that hemp oil was popular because it could be used for other aspects of life. Unlike marijuana, hemp oil has low levels of THC and doesn't have psychoactive properties.

Although the whole hemp plant is used to produce it, usually seeds are the parts that give the best oil.

What most people don't know is that hemp oil is an excellent source of the omega-6 and omega-3 fatty acids that our body needs to function properly.

Today, hemp oil is praised for having these health benefits:

- maintains hormonal balance in the body
- energizes and rejuvenates skin
- great sources of omega-3s and omega-6s for vegetarians
- lowers cholesterol

Beneficial for diabetes:

- prevents psoriasis
- boosts immunity
- prevents varicose veins

Hemp and Hemp Oil Throughout History: A Timeline

We already know that hemp oil has many health benefits (just like marijuana), but it is also used for skincare, textile production, building materials, foods, flours, and oils. Hemp homes have even been constructed.

Let's review the timeline regarding the most important historical events surrounding hemp and hemp oil.

- 8000 BC—Hemp is used in Taiwan for fiber and for food. Also, production of hemp accounts for one of the oldest industries. For example, the oldest relic of human industry is a piece of hemp fabric that dates back to 8000 BC and was found in Mesopotamia. Assyrian scripts also mention hemp industry.
- 3000 BC—Hemp is used for medical purposes in China and Taiwan. By this time, it is also considered as the most important textile, even in China (it was cheaper than silk and was used to clothe the peasants). Throughout the years it has been used in war-related articles because of its enormous strength, e.g. bow strings and naval ropes.
- 2000 BC—Ancient Egyptians use hemp for medical purposes and clothing.
- 2000–1400 BC—Vedic writings embrace cannabis as a source of happiness and joy. It is valued for its ability to eliminate fear.
- 700 BC—Scythians use hemp oil to purify and cleanse themselves.

The Anti-Aging Miracles of Hemp-Derived CBD Oil

- 700–600 BC—The Zoroastrian *Zend-Avesta* is written and refers to bhang, or cannabis, as the "good narcotic."
- 600 BC—Hemp rope appears in southern Russia.
- 500 BC—The Scythians introduce hemp to Europe where its use spreads.
- 100 BC—Hemp is turned into paper in China.
- 23-79—Pliny the Elder documents hemp rope and analgesic effects.
- 130-200—Greek physician Galen prescribes medical marijuana.
- 850—The Vikings bring hemp rope and seeds to Iceland.
- 900—Arabs use hemp paper.
- 1400s—Christopher Columbus carries hemp seeds on his ships, planning to plant the seeds in case of shipwreck in order to grow raw materials for supplies and for food.
- 1533—King Henry VIII fines farmers who do not grow hemp.
- 1776—The Declaration of Independence was signed on hemp paper.
- 1790s—George Washington, Thomas Jefferson, and John Adams grow hemp.
- 1800s—Until this period, the term *linen* was used to describe any fabric made from hemp.
- 1840s—Abraham Lincoln uses hemp oil as fuel for lamps in his household.
- 1942–1946—Farmers in the U.S. harvest more than 150,000 acres of hemp through the USDA's "Hemp for Victory" program.
- 1986—The Chernobyl Nuclear Plant reactor in Ukraine causes severe radioactive contamination. Industrial hemp is used for phyto-remediation.[7]
- 1998—The US legalizes the import of hemp oil and food-grade hemp seed.
    (www.triplepundit.com/2011/05/hemp-history-week-pushes-legalizing-industrial-hemp-usa/)

---

[7] Phyto-remediation is the process of using plants to remove contaminants from the soil.

- 2001—The DEA publishes a press release in October of 2001, banning all hemp seed and oil food products (even without THC). The hemp seed industry is in a quandary as no detection protocol for THC is specified. Furthermore, while poppy seeds (from which opiates are derived) are alright, non-psychoactive hemp is not.
- 2003—The struggle continues over the status of hemp, but regardless of different statutes and laws, it is illegal to import hemp oil and seeds thereby making it impossible to manufacture or sell any hemp products. The Hemp Industries Association files an Urgent Motion for Stay in the 9th Circuit Court of Appeals.
- 2004—The Ninth Circuit Court reaches a decision in favor of the Hemp Industries Association, protecting the sale of hemp-containing foods. Hemp remains legal for import and sale, even though farmers are still not permitted to grow it.
- 2014—Congress enacts The Agricultural Act, also known as 2014 Farm Bill. It allows state departments of agriculture to grow and cultivate industrial hemp for medical and research purposes only. Furthermore, each state has to allow this cultivation. The act paves the way for legalization of CBD oil.

The Anti-Aging Miracles of Hemp-Derived CBD Oil

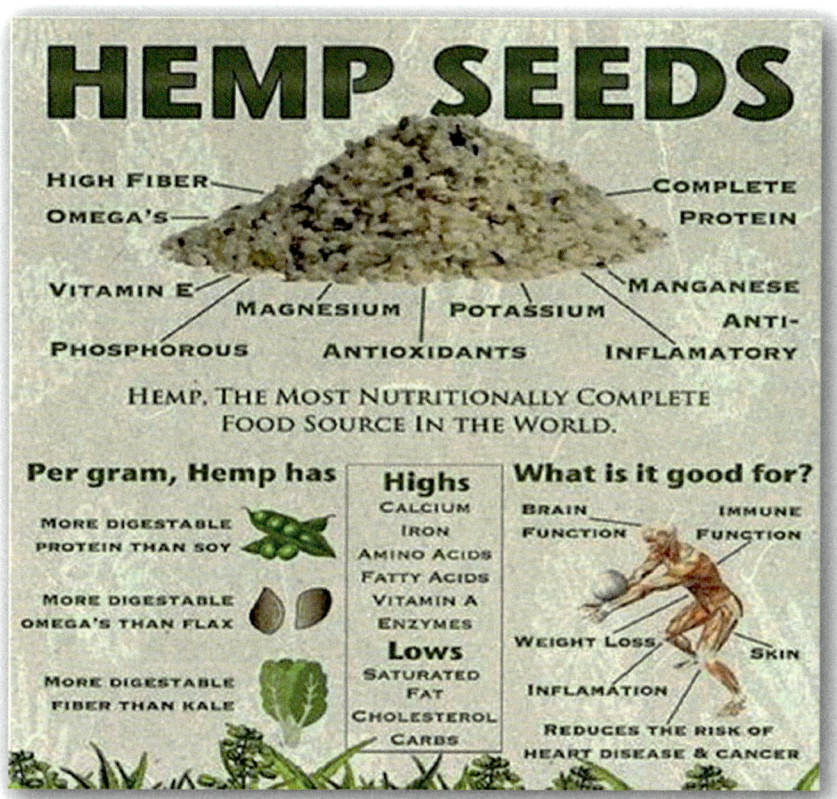

Hemp seeds' benefits infographic (courtesy of evohemp.com)

CHAPTER 6

Health Benefits of Marijuana and Hemp Success Stories

ALTHOUGH THE PRODUCTION of marijuana or even hemp is severely forbidden by the law, patients are able to obtain medical marijuana in some parts of the world to help relieve pain or symptoms connected with diseases. The benefits of marijuana are well documented throughout history, but they're still subjected to ongoing debates among scientists. While some scientists dismiss any claims about health benefits, describing marijuana as a mere drug, others firmly believe that their beneficial effects on one's health are unquestionable.

In this chapter, we'll take a closer look at marijuana and hemp success stories to demonstrate how one seemingly simple plant can make a person's life much better.

Story 1: Marijuana stops child's severe seizures

By most standards, Paige and Matt Figi had it all. They lived the American dream. The couple met at Colorado State University, got married, and had a baby boy, who they named Max. When their son was two, the couple decided to have another baby, and their happiness went through the roof when Paige got pregnant with twins. Chase and Charlotte were born on October 18, 2006. Both babies seemed perfectly healthy when they were born.

The Anti-Aging Miracles of Hemp-Derived CBD Oil

The twins were only three months old when troubles began. Charlotte had just had a bath, and Matt was putting on her diaper. "She was lying on her back on the floor," said Matt, "and her eyes just started flickering."

The baby's seizure lasted about half an hour. The frightened parents rushed her daughter to the hospital immediately.

"They weren't calling it epilepsy. We just thought it was one random seizure. They did a $1 million work-up—the MRI, EEG, spinal tap. They did the whole workup and found nothing and sent us home," Paige said.

However, just seven days later, Charlotte experienced another seizure. This time, the seizure was longer and marked the beginning of frequent seizures that Charlotte experienced over the next few months. Some seizures lasted up to two hours.

Doctors were puzzled because the baby's blood tests were perfectly normal, just like the scans she had undergone.

Only when the baby was two-and-a-half years old did the doctors successfully determine the diagnosis. Charlotte suffered from Dravet syndrome. The syndrome is, in fact, a rare and severe intractable form of epilepsy ("intractable" means that seizures experienced by patients cannot be controlled with medications). The first seizures in Dravet syndrome occur before the age of one. In the second year, other seizures appear, such as involuntary muscle spasms.

Paige took her toddler to the Dravet expert in Chicago, who recommended a ketogenic diet, which is known for relieving seizures associated with epilepsy. The diet helped manage Charlotte's seizures, but it came with various side effects, such as bone loss and weakened immune system.

Matt constantly tried to find new ways online to help her daughter, and at some point he found a video of a boy from California whose seizures in Dravet syndrome were successfully treated with cannabis. By that time, Charlotte had lost the ability to walk, eat, and talk. Even the little girl's heart stopped on numerous occasions. When she was five, doctors in the hospital told Matt and Paige that there was nothing they could do about their daughter's disease anymore. That's when Paige decided to try medical marijuana.

Charlotte was the youngest patient in Colorado to apply for medical marijuana. Paige admitted it wasn't easy to find a doctor who would prescribe it. The main issue for all doctors was the fact that Charlotte was just a child and, although marijuana proved to be beneficial for various health conditions, it wasn't quite clear how it would affect a child.

Then, Paige reached Dr. Margaret Gedde who agreed to meet the family. The family also contacted Dr. Alan Shackelford. She said, "They had exhausted all of her treatment options. There really weren't any steps they could take beyond what they had done. Everything had been tried—except cannabis."

Paige found a dispensary in Denver and paid $800 for two ounces of medical marijuana, which was extracted into oil. First, they started with small doses. Page wrote, "When she didn't have those three, four seizures that first hour, that was the first sign, and I thought well, 'Let's go another hour, this has got to be a fluke…

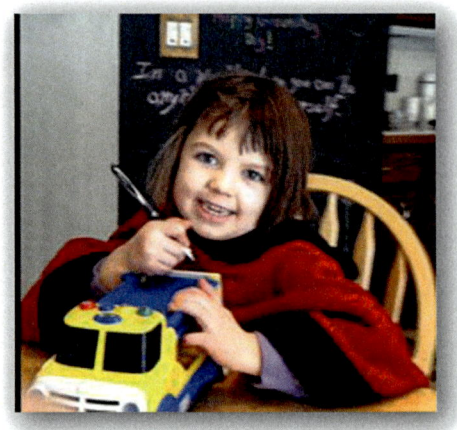

Image courtesy of http://asa-nc.com/

But the seizures completely stopped for an entire week."

However, the supply of marijuana for the little girl was running out. Paige then heard about the Stanley brothers, who were one of the largest marijuana growers in the state. When they heard about the girl's age, they were skeptical, but once they met Charlotte, the brothers were on board.

Matt and Paige can't hide their happiness and excitement regarding how beneficial marijuana has been for their daughter. Now, Charlotte experiences seizures three to four times a month and usually in her sleep instead of constantly during the day. Not only is Charlotte walking, but she also rides her bike, talks,6 laughs, and feeds herself. The marijuana strain that helps Charlotte and many other pediatric epileptic patients is called "Charlotte's Web," after this little girl who got her life back. The story was reported by CNN.

The Anti-Aging Miracles of Hemp-Derived CBD Oil

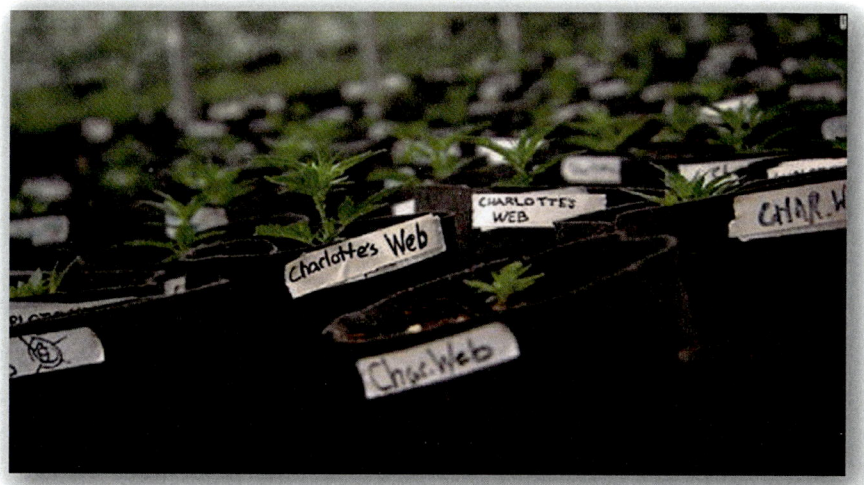

Charlotte's Web (photo courtesy of CW Botanicals)

Story 2: Marijuana helps one woman overcome cachexia

Shona Banda was diagnosed with Crohn's disease in 2004. She underwent a series of surgeries and had to take a wide range of medications. However, instead of feeling better, Shona's condition started to worsen progressively.

Shona was bedridden and began suffering from cachexia,[8] which often accompanies Crohn's disease. Shona's condition was so severe that she virtually waited to die. Luckily, she heard about *Rick Simpson's Run from the Cure* video documentary and was inspired to try marijuana.

However, Shona didn't have enough marijuana to make oils to treat her condition as discussed by Simpson. So, she started inhaling small amounts of marijuana from a vaporizer just to reduce the pain and improve her impaired appetite.

---

[8] Cachexia is weakness and wasting of the body due to severe chronic condition.

Shona's husband then noted something that would prove to be extremely beneficial for his wife's health—the marijuana vapor residue inside the glass globe cover looked like marijuana oil. Shona started scraping the oil and putting it into capsules for consumption. She took these capsules three times a day.

After just a few days, Shona was able to get up and walk without a cane, which was unimaginable before. Her health significantly improved. Her appetite improved and her sleeping pattern improved as well.

Shona's story about surviving Crohn's disease and cachexia was published on YouTube: https://www.youtube.com/watch?v=x_otUB7pVMA.

Story 3: Marijuana reduces essential tremor symptoms and tremor associated with Parkinson's disease

Marijuana is believed to have beneficial effects on one's brain. For example, it's associated with slowing down dementia and Alzheimer's disease and also with reducing symptoms of Parkinson's disease.

An example of using marijuana to reduce tremors linked with Parkinson's disease is that of the famous actor Michael J. Fox. Fox first developed symptoms of this disease when he was only twenty-nine years old and was actually diagnosed with Parkinson's disease at the age of thirty-seven. Fox admitted that using cannabis helped him ease the symptoms of Parkinson's disease and reduce tremors.

Let's move on to essential tremor. It's a nervous system disorder that causes rhythmic shaking. It can affect any part of person's body, but it usually occurs in a person's hands. Medical marijuana has been known to help reduce the intensity and severity of tremors. Many tremor sufferers have reported personal experiences in which marijuana proves beneficial for their condition. On the flip side, marijuana loosens muscles to prevent spasticity and uncontrollable movements.

The Anti-Aging Miracles of Hemp-Derived CBD Oil

Story 4: Marijuana reduces vomiting and nausea in complicated pregnancy

Some pregnant women diagnosed with *hyperemesis gravidarum* have found relief in marijuana. Hyperemesis gravidarum is essentially a severe morning sickness in early pregnancy

Zahra was a pregnant woman with hyperemesis gravidarum who found relief in medical marijuana. When she found out she was pregnant, Zahra was ecstatic. To celebrate her pregnancy, Zahra went out to eat, only to vomit intensely shortly after her meal.

She suffered from severe nausea and vomiting for three months. She lost all her strength and couldn't even walk or eat. Luckily, Zahra gave birth to a perfectly normal little girl.

Eventually, she joined the navy, where she met her current husband. Soon, they decided to have a baby and conceived easily. However, her troubles started with intense vomiting. She was incapacitated with the vomiting. Again she couldn't walk, eat, or do anything. Zahra even had thoughts of abortion. Luckily, she admits, she found marijuana.

The retching and vomiting were controlled, and she was able to eat better. She regained the pounds she lost and became an avid supporter for legalizing medical marijuana.

Story 5: Woman beats lung cancer with cannabis oil

When a fifty-four-year-old wife and mother, Sharon Kelly, started experiencing sharp pains on the left side of her body near her ribs, she thought it was related to a strong massage she had had that day. However, after several days without relief, Sharon thought the problem was something other than just a massage. And she was right.

Sally Schutz, M.D. & Bayne Boyes, FCPA

She visited her health care provider, who found that Sharon had lung cancer. In just a few weeks, the prognosis worsened. She was told that the cancer in her body affected her lymph nodes and the lining of her stomach. She only had six to nine months to live.

Sharon asked the doctors about possible treatments, including chemotherapy or radiation, but was told that given the size of the cancer, these treatments simply wouldn't work.

Doctors had given up on her when Sharon's youngest daughter conducted some research on the Internet. She found a number of testimonials of cancer survivors who reported that marijuana had helped them beat cancer. Sharon started taking cannabis oil in small dosages a few times a day.

Eventually, Sharon upped her dosage and after a few months of regular consumption, her tumor shrank from 5 cm to 2.1, and her lymph nodes retained their normal size. Seven months after her treatment with cannabis oil, Sharon was declared cancer-free.

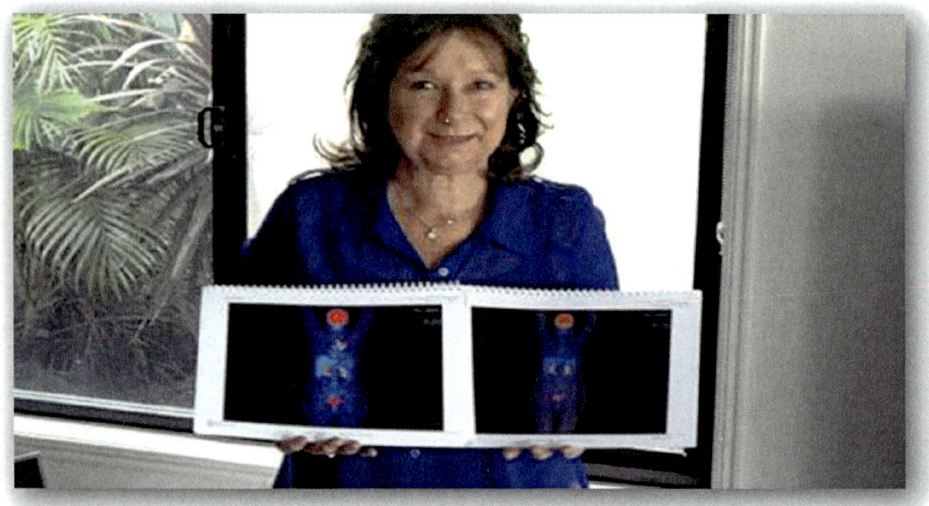

Image courtesy of www.cureyourowncancer.org

Story 6: Marijuana cures insomnia

Pain News Network published testimonials of people who have used marijuana to treat different health issues. One was given by a schoolteacher who prefers to be anonymous. The individual suffered from Ehlers-Danlos syndrome, an inherited disorder that affects a person's connective tissues, primarily the skin, joints, and blood vessel walls. This woman also had intractable insomnia.

Due to her disease and inability to fall asleep, the schoolteacher couldn't perform her job well. She decided to try medical marijuana, or more precisely cannabis oil, every night before bedtime.

Cannabis oil didn't only help her sleep, but it also relieved the pain she felt within ten minutes of taking each dose.

Story 7: ALS patient benefits from smoking cannabis

In 1985, Cathy Jordan started experiencing difficulty with her basic motor skills: she had trouble picking things up. A year later, she was diagnosed with Amyotrophic Lateral Sclerosis (ALS), [9] and doctors gave her only three years to live.

In the late 1980s, Cathy started treating herself with marijuana and felt better! However, when she informed her doctors that she was using an illegal substance to treat her condition, many of them reacted with a prohibitionist mindset and without compassion.

She recalled, "I visited a neurologist at Duke University, and when I told him that I was smoking cannabis, he didn't really know what to do with me. The doctor was afraid. He didn't even want to take my blood pressure because I was using an illegal substance."

---

9 Amyotrophic Lateral Sclerosis (ALS) is a progressive neurological condition that affects the muscular motor function of the limbs and vital organs. It affects 30,000 Americans.

Cathy's health care providers didn't want to accept the fact that she was better because of marijuana and that the plant managed to extend her lifespan. She also reported that some doctors threatened that they'd have her committed because what she was doing was simply illegal.

In 2012, Cathy recalled, "All my doctors are either dead or retiring. I have outlived five support groups and four different neurologists."

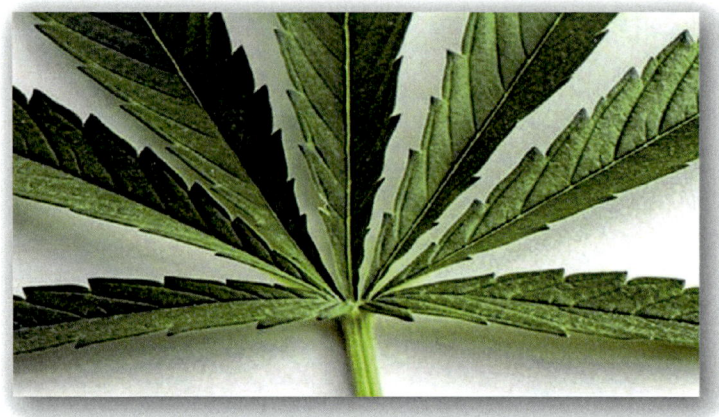

Image courtesy of Boltenkoff:*shutterstock.com*

Summary

The Marijuana Tax Act of 1937 made possession of marijuana illegal throughout the United States. The act excluded industrial and medical uses, but the government imposed an excise tax on all sales of hemp.

Annual fees ranged from $1 to $24 depending on the classification as a professional; non –professional or manufacturer, importer etc. respectively; basically the main purpose of annul fees was to enforce registration. Transaction fees were $1/oz for those registered and $100/oz for non-registrants.

The American Medical Association opposed this decision, mostly because the taxes were imposed on health care providers who prescribed cannabis. The government of the United States proceeded to pass this act because of poorly attended hearings and cannabis reports based on questionable studies opposed by the AMA.

Basically, the federal government was convinced that marijuana wasn't beneficial for one's health; in fact, the government thought that cannabis could only cause addiction. Thousands of patient testimonials continue to prove otherwise.

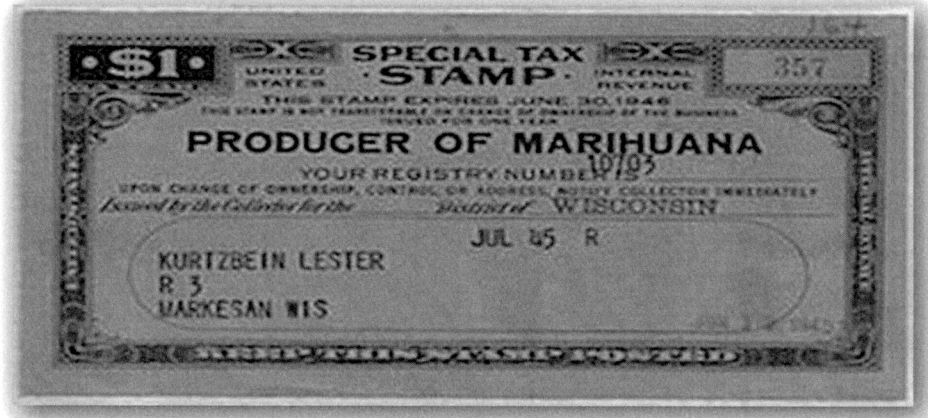

Tax stamp for marijuana (courtesy of henak.com)

CHAPTER 7

Cannabinoid Patent

ALTHOUGH CANNABIS HAS been used in medical practices for thousands of years and its benefits are confirmed by thousands of people worldwide, the usage of this plant is still quite limited. Yes, various U.S. states and some other countries legalized the usage of medical marijuana, but that's still not enough if you take into account the global scale. It's not only the problem of psychoactive properties and fear that people would use it as a recreational drug. There is also the patent issue.

Herbs and plants, as well as herbal medicines and formulas, generally can't be patented. Therefore, there is not enough financial incentive to explore the properties and possibilities of these plants. Without enough clinical studies, research, and data, there's simply no basis for knowing whether these plants could match medical standards today.

Furthermore, patents usually rely on the ability to recognize and identify a certain active agent. On the other hand, traditional herbology systems refer to the synergy of a wide range of herbs to achieve desired results. This synergy is complicated and almost impossible to prove with scientific methods.

The primary reason why a wide range of plants and herbs aren't used for treatments of various diseases (although they're quite beneficial) is because the inability to patent these plants makes them essentially worthless for pharmaceutical companies.

When a pharmaceutical company holds a patent for a certain formula, it allows the company to profit. Since they cannot patent the plant or herb, nothing stops other pharmaceutical companies or even governments from using that plant for their own purposes.

The lack of clinical studies regarding the benefits of cannabis is one of the reasons for the absence of corporate or government interest. This causes a domino effect, e.g. no clinical research, no scientifically confirmed benefits, no production, no accessibility of the plant to all people who would benefit from it.

Marijuana Patent Belongs to...

Although the U.S. government spokespeople consistently have pointed out that marijuana doesn't have any healing properties, the shocking reality is that the U.S. holds the patent to the components of cannabis known as cannabinoids.

Patent No. 6630507 is held by the Department of Health and Human Services and covers the use of cannabinoids for treating a wide range of diseases. The patent is entitled "Cannabinoids as Antioxidants and Neuroprotectants." It was awarded to the U.S. government on October 7, 2003. Imagine! Exclusive rights held by this patent refer to the usage of cannabinoids for:

- Alzheimer's disease
- Parkinson's disease
- diseases caused by oxidative stress
- stroke
- heart attack
- Crohn's disease
- arthritis
- diabetes

Sally Schutz, M.D. & Bayne Boyes, FCPA

(12) **United States Patent** (10) Patent No.: **US 6,630,507 B1**
Hampson et al. (45) Date of Patent: **Oct. 7, 2003**

(54) CANNABINOIDS AS ANTIOXIDANTS AND NEUROPROTECTANTS

(75) Inventors: **Aidan J. Hampson**, Irvine, CA (US); **Julius Axelrod**, Rockville, MD (US); **Maurizio Grimaldi**, Bethesda, MD (US)

(73) Assignee: **The United States of America as represented by the Department of Health and Human Services**, Washington, DC (US)

(*) Notice: Subject to any disclaimer, the term of this

OTHER PUBLICATIONS

Windholz et al., The Merck Index, Tenth Edition (1983) p. 241, abstract No. 1723.*
Mechoulam et al., "A Total Synthesis of dl–Δ^1–Tetrahydrocannabinol, the Active Constituent of Hashish[1]," *Journal of the American Chemical Society*, 87:14:3273–3275 (1965).
Mechoulam et al., "Chemical Basis of Hashish Activity," *Science*, 18:611–612 (1970).
Ottersen et al., "The Crystal and Molecular Structure of Cannabidiol," *Acta Chem. Scand. B 31*, 9:807–812 (1977).
Cunha et al., "Chronic Administration of Cannabidiol to Healthy Volunteers and Epileptic Patients[1]," *Pharmacology,*

Patent 6630507

According to the patent, the primary aim is to provide a whole new class of *antioxidant drugs* that have particular use as *neuroprotectants*. Another intent is to provide a class of drugs that are *non-psychoactive*, "non-toxic even at very high doses and have *good tissue penetration*, for example crossing the blood brain barrier."

The patent does not include THC.

CHAPTER 8

Discovery of the Endocannabinoid System by Dr. R. Mechoulam

I HAVE ALREADY mentioned Dr. Mechoulam in chapter three. In this chapter, we'll discuss some of his amazing contributions to medical science.

Who is Dr. Raphael Mechoulam?

Raphael Mechoulam was born in 1930 in Sofia, Bulgaria. He is a well-known organic chemist and a professor of medicinal chemistry at the Hebrew University of Jerusalem.

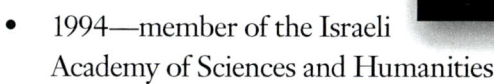

He is best known for his work in the isolation of THC and many other studies that involve cannabis.

For research, Dr. Mechoulam (photo courtesy of phytec.com) received numerous honors, including:

- 1994—member of the Israeli Academy of Sciences and Humanities
- 2000—Israel Prize in Exact Sciences (chemistry)
- 2001—Ohio State University honorary doctorate
- 2002—honorary member of the Israel Society of Psychology and Pharmacology

- 2006—Compultense University of Madrid honorary doctorate
- 2011—NIDA discovery award
- 2012—EMET Prize in Exact Sciences—Chemistry

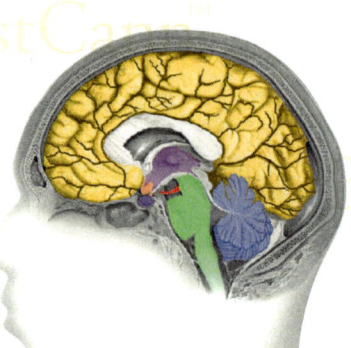

Image Courtesy of BestCann CBD Oil

What is the Endocannabinoid System?

The endocannabinoid system (ECS) is defined as a central regulatory system that affects various biological processes. The system consists of a group of molecules that are called cannabinoids and cannabinoid receptors to which these molecules attach.

Even though cannabis is known as a source of more than 111 cannabinoids (out of which THC is the most "famous" one), our body produces a significant amount of cannabinoids as well.

The Anti-Aging Miracles of Hemp-Derived CBD Oil

After decades of scientific studies, two cannabinoid receptors have been identified:

- CB1
- CB2

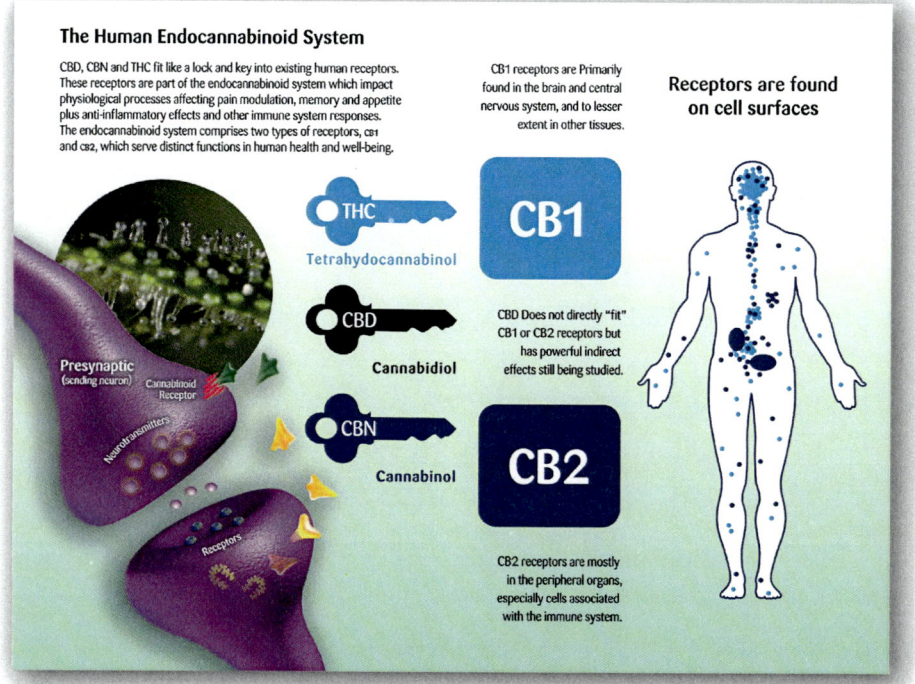

The human endocannabinoid system (courtesy of medicinalgenomics.com)

Let's look at some of the systems in our body with CB1 or CB2 receptors:

- gastrointestinal system
- cardiovascular system
- reproductive system
- urinary system
- immune system
- nervous system (including the brain)

What do these cannabinoid receptors actually do? Well, they act as binding sites or attaching points for endogenous cannabinoids (that is, cannabinoid substances our own bodies make), just like cannabinoids from the plant. When these cannabinoids attach to CB1 or CB2, they change the way the body functions.

What is the Purpose of the Endocannabinoid System?

The endocannabinoid system isn't unique to humans. Several studies show that mammals, like horses, cats, dogs, and pigs as well as non-mammals, have endocannabinoid systems and receptors.

Even though the ECS has a big impact on a series of biological processes, experts believe its primary role is the regulation of *homeostasis*. This process is essential for all living beings, and it is defined as the body's ability to maintain stable internal conditions that are necessary to survive.

This is so important it bears repeating: *The ECS is the master control system that balances the body.*

Ailments and illnesses are in fact consequences of the inability to achieve homeostasis. Any desire to maintain health and well-being, to bulletproof your health, to promote an anti-aging regimen, requires strengthening the endocannabinoid system.

Life's stresses and toxins cause an imbalance in the ECS, which is why supporting the ECS with external cannabinoids, like hemp-derived CBD oil, has caught the eye of bio-hacking enthusiasts.

Dr. Mechoulam has been investigating this system longer than any other scientist. He defines the endocannabinoid system as a "supercomputer that regulates homeostasis in the human body." *Because receptors are*

The Anti-Aging Miracles of Hemp-Derived CBD Oil

found in the brain as well as other parts of the body, it is believed that an imbalance in this system is implicated in most disease states.

Furthermore, Dr. Mechoulam has indicated time and time again that the importance of the endocannabinoid system for homeostasis is also a primary reason why cannabis affects a broad range of diseases and health issues, from glaucoma to cancer, from seizures to vomiting. He has investigated the role of cannabis in the treatment of schizophrenia and PTSD.

The ECS is even triggered at birth when the infant suckles at the breast, receiving cannabinoids in the breast milk. The genius of this system allows for the bonding of the baby to its mother at the same time that it is receiving calming cannabinoids.

For his contributions in defining and being at the forefront of cannabinoid research, Dr. Mechoulam is universally acknowledged as the father of cannabinoid science.

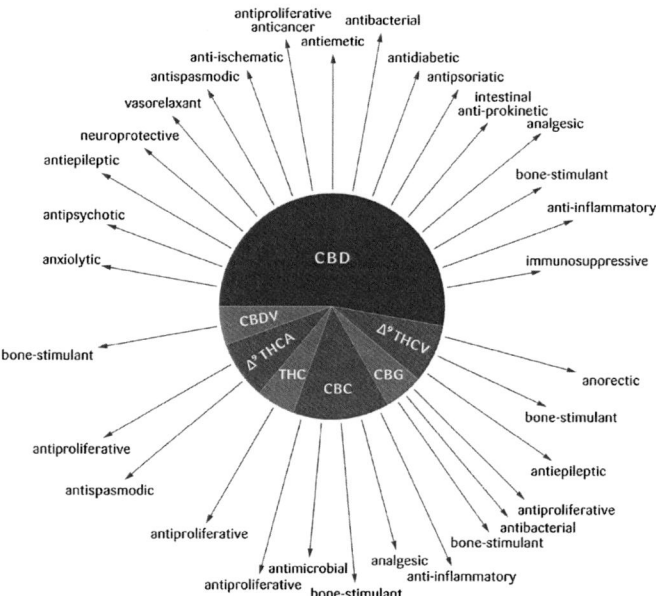

Image Courtesy of BestCann.com

Now that we know what the endocannabinoid system is and why it's important for our body and overall health, let's take a closer look at the systems it affects.

The Endocannabinoid System and Bones

Itai Bab, from the Bone Laboratory at the Hebrew University of Jerusalem, conducted several studies to determine the link between the endocannabinoid system and our bones.

In his most recent study, whose findings were published in the *British Journal of Pharmacology* (January, 2008), Itai Bab pointed out that the endocannabinoid system has an important role in the regulation of skeletal remodeling and the consequent implications of bone mass, as well as biochemical function.

A team of scientists, led by Bab, has identified the CB1 cannabinoid receptor in sympathetic terminals innervating the skeleton. They have stressed the importance of further studies to observe and investigate the role of the CB1 receptor in bone turnover, as well as the role of the CB2 cannabinoid receptor found in bone cells. Genetic research indicating errors in certain genes that regulate the CB2 receptors may provide a genetic risk factor for osteoporosis.

This study is of huge importance because the notion that our bones have cannabinoid receptors suggests that the use of hemp-derived cannabinoid oil can significantly impact bone health in a positive way.

The Endocannabinoid System and Inflammation of the Joints

Due to its anti-inflammatory properties, endocannabinoids reduce the pain associated with arthritis. The team of Dr. D. Richardson at the

British Center for Analytical Bioscience published a study in the journal *Arthritis Research and Therapy* (April, 2008).

Thirty-two participants diagnosed with osteoarthritis and thirteen participants with rheumatoid arthritis were studied. The findings suggested that cannabinoids are present in the synovia, the soft tissue of joints of osteoarthritis and rheumatoid arthritis patients. The research suggested that cannabinoid receptors present in the soft tissue of many joints could be an important therapeutic target for the treatment of pain and inflammation associated arthritis. Again, the use of hemp-derived cannabinoid oil seems to reduce inflammation associated with different forms of arthritis.

This bears repeating: the endocannabinoid system could be one of the body's natural mechanisms for combating arthritis.

The Endocannabinoid System and the Brain

The endocannabinoid system is different from other neurotransmitter systems. For example, endocannabinoids act as modulators that inhibit the release of other neurotransmitters like gamma-aminobutyric acid (GABA)[10] and glutamate.[11]

Simplistically, the endocannabinoids are involved in what is called, signaling retrogrades.[12] They are released from the presynaptic (sending) neuron, as well as the postsynaptic neuron synthesizes where endocannabinoids are further released into the synaptic clef. This is depicted in the image below:

---

10 GABA is the main inhibitory neurotransmitter in the central nervous system.
11 Glutamate is the major mediator of excitatory signals in the central nervous system.
12 Endocannabinoid signaling has been implicated in learning and memory, specifically in extinction of aversive memories (http://www.ncbi.nlm.nih.gov/pmc/articles/PMC1352167/).

Sally Schutz, M.D. & Bayne Boyes, FCPA

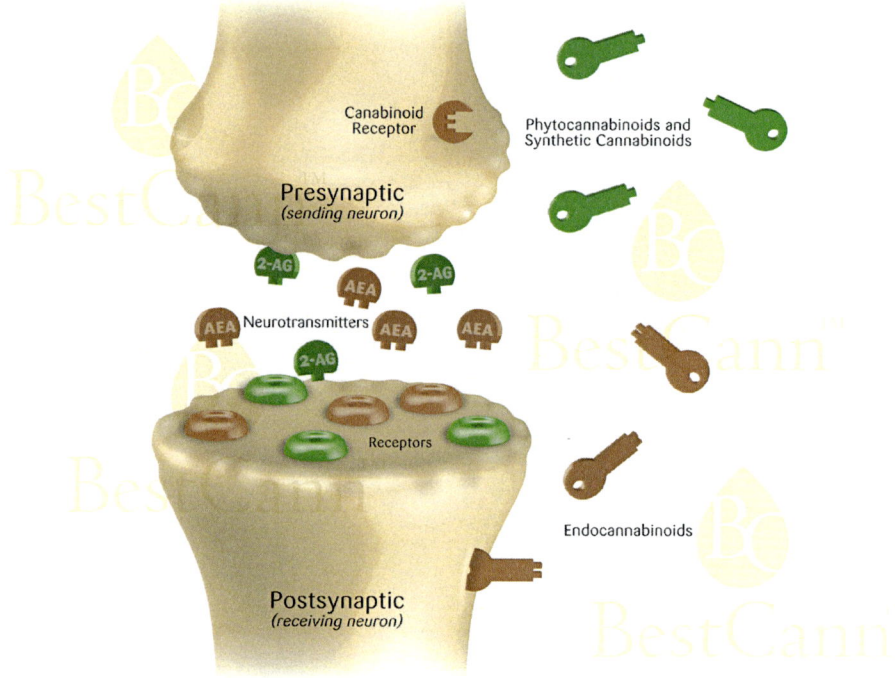

Endocannabinoids are unique, they travel in the both directions and deliver feedback to the presynaptic cell (courtesy of bestcann.com).

Considering that research on the endocannabinoid system is in its infancy and that the brain is considered to be the organ with the highest number of cannabinoid receptors, scientists continue to investigate the importance of the endocannabinoid system on our brain and its relevance to maintaining health, reversing disease, as well as it importance in anti-aging.

The Anti-Aging Miracles of Hemp-Derived CBD Oil

Dr. Esther Shohami, from The Institute of Drug Research at Faculty of Medicine of the Hebrew University of Jerusalem, is known for her studies that observe the link between the endocannabinoid system, the brain, and brain injuries.

Dr. Shohami has published results of her studies in many notable medical journals, including the *British Journal of Pharmacology*. Among her most important discoveries are:

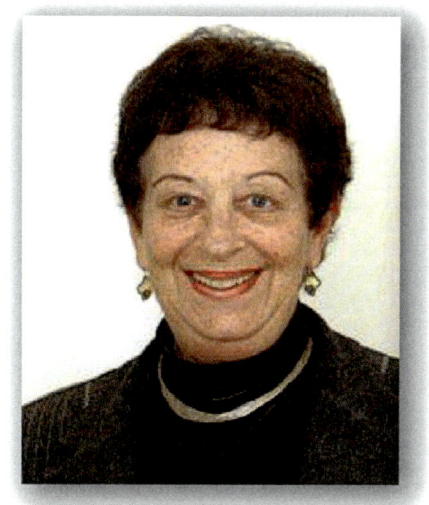

Dr Esther Shohami courtesy of estyshohami.ekmd.huji.ac.il

- Unlike standard neurotransmitters, endocannabinoids aren't stored in presynaptic vesicles. In fact, they are produced "on demand."
- Endocannabinoids interact with at least three types of receptors at binding sites located in different parts of the brain.
- The interaction between endocannabinoids and receptors depends on a wide range of factors, such as levels of endocannabinoids, distribution of tissue receptors, and accessibility to these receptors.
- Neuronal injury activates endocannabinoid signaling as an *intrinsic neuroprotective* response by activating signaling pathways downstream from cannabinoid receptors. This promotes neuronal function and maintenance.
- Activation of CB2 receptors by synthetic specific agonists provides *neuroprotection* in ischemic stroke.

Shohami's studies are important because they elucidate the role of the endocannabinoid system in brain health and brain injuries. While research continues to look for new opportunities to tackle and successfully reverse various traumatic brain injuries, hemp-derived CBD can be utilized to help stabilize and protect the central nervous system.

Accumulation of these mediators leads to neuro-inflammation, cell death, and vasoconstriction and culminates in secondary damage. When this happens, there is also an on-demand production of endocannabinoids to inhibit excitotoxicity damage to act as antioxidants and to counteract vasoconstrictor effects. Then endocannabinoids augment stem cells. A critical function of endocannabinoids is to reduce secondary damage, thus acting as endogenous neuroprotectants.

As seen on the schematic representation below, a brain injury leads to the release of harmful mediators that accumulate in the brain.

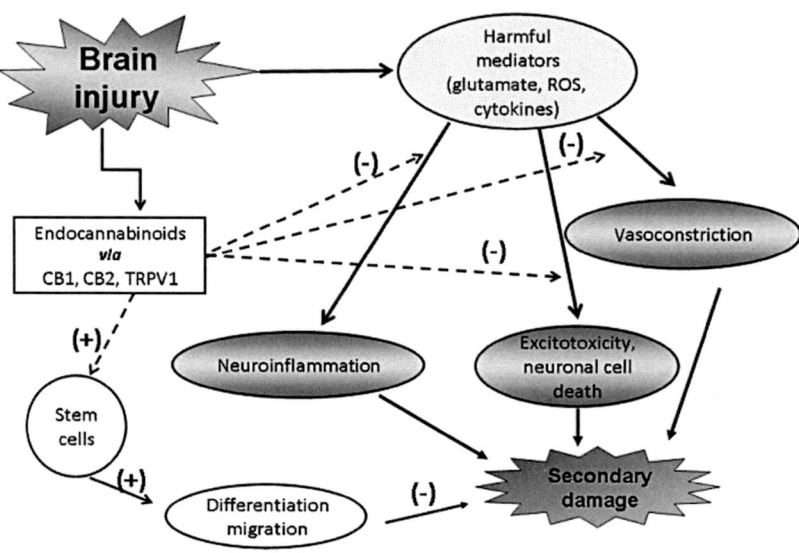

Schematic representation of Dr. Shohami's research on brain injury (courtesy of http://www.ncbi.nlm.nih.gov/pmc/articles/PMC3165950)

The Endocannabinoid System and Immunity

Endocannabinoids have complex regulatory effects on the immune system involving innate, humoral and cell mediated immunity. The cannabinoids affect apoptosis (cell death), cytokines, and T-regulatory cells (Braun et al *Immunobiology*, April 2011). The effects of cannabinoids on the immune system appear to be more pronounced under stressful conditions, and their protective role against tissue damage is being elucidated (Pacher and Mechoulam *Progress in Lipid Research*, February 2011).

The importance of the role of the endocannabinoid system in regulating homeostasis, modulating our immune system, and reducing inflammation (thereby keeping us healthy), cannot be over emphasized.

Phytocannabinoids strengthen the endocannabinoid system by improving the response from immune signaling in two ways: by anti-inflammatory actions and by stimulating our cannabinoid receptors (http://www.whale.to/a/human5.html). This serves to improve health, suggesting various therapeutic effects including:

- reduction of seizures in epilepsy
- anti-nausea and appetite improvement
- insulin sensitivity
- improvement of sleep
- pain relief (particularly chronic)
- decreased intensity and severity of autoimmune and inflammatory diseases

The Endocannabinoid System and Inflammation in the Body

Both cannabinoid receptors, CB1 and CB2, contain high levels of neurons, as well as central and peripheral immune cells. Both receptors regulate inflammation, thereby affecting the central nervous system (http://www.ncbi.nlm.nih.gov/pmc/articles/PMC4070159/), degenerative diseases, and other systemic diseases. Research by Professor Emeritus Ruth Gallily at the Hebrew University of Jerusalem has studied the promising anti-inflammatoryproperties of cannabis in arthritis (http://www.researchgate.net/publication/281053965-_HU444_A_Novel_Potent_Anti-Inflammatory_Non-Psychotropic_Cannabinoid).

The Endocannabinoid System and Cardiovascular Benefits

Rosen et al in the American Journal of Physiology, Hearth and Circulatory Physiology (Ronen et al: Am J Physiol Heart Circ Physiol 293: H3602–H3607, 2007) describe their research on cannabis and the cardiovascular system.

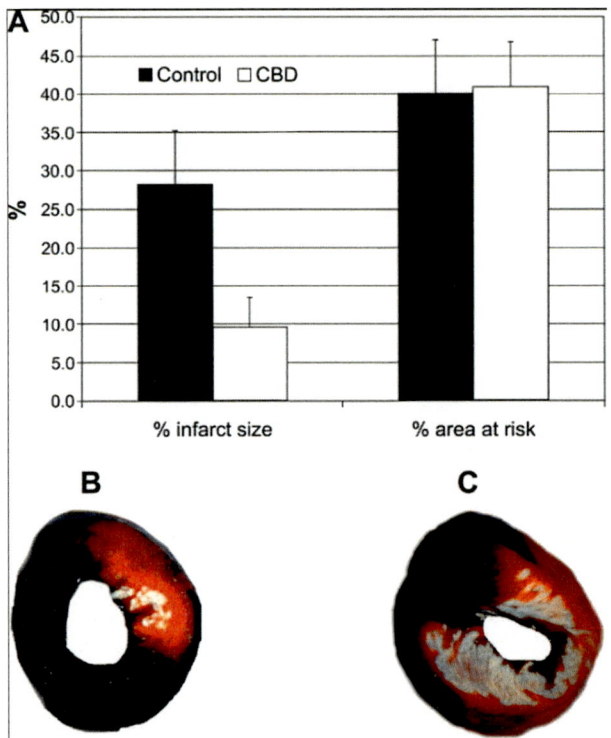

Cannabis helps repair damage and promotes recovery after heart attacks. The photo above shows the consequences of cardiac damage (exhibit C) and the remarkable effects of the treatment with cannabis (exhibit B).

Endocannabinoid System and Diabetes

Compelling evidence from a number of different studies suggests that the endocannabinoid system inhibits diabetes-caused oxidative stress and inflammation. Dr. Gallily who was mentioned above shows promising results with cannabis and diabetes (http://www.israel21c.org/cannabis-extract-to-be-used-to-treat-diabetes/).

Animal studies by Weiss et al (http://www.ncbi.nlm.nih.gov/-pmc/articles-/PMC2270485/) showed cannabidiol arrested the onset of autoimmune diabetes in non-obese diabetic mice. Cannabidiol actually lowered the incidence of diabetes in young non-obese diabetes prone female mice. In human studies at the Harvard School of Public Health, cannabinoids were found to aid in regulating insulin in the blood (http://www.amjmed.com/article/S0002-9343(13)00200-3/abstract). Cannabinoid research is proliferating in the field of diabetes and metabolic balance.

The American Alliance for Medical Cannabis provides information indicating that cannabis helps:

- stabilize blood sugars
- suppress some of the arterial inflammation commonly experienced by diabetics, which can lead to cardiovascular disease
- prevent nerve inflammation and ease the pain of neuropathy (a common complication of diabetes)
- lower blood pressure over time (this can help reduce the risk of heart disease [*European Journal of Nutrition August* 2014, Volume 53, Issue 5, pp 1,237–1,246]).
- keep blood vessels open and improve circulation
- relieve muscle cramps and the pain of gastrointestinal disorders
- relieve neuropathic pain and tingling in hands and feet (think diabetic neuropathy)

The Endocannabinoid System and Phantom Limb Pain

Phantom limb pain refers to an ongoing painful sensation that seems to be coming from a limb that is no longer there and is frequent in patients who have had their arms or legs amputated.

Cannabinoids are regarded as beneficial for phantom limb pain (http://-www.ncbi.nlm.nih.gov/pmc/articles/PMC2430692/).

The Endocannabinoid System and PTSD

The huge importance of the endocannabinoid system goes beyond our physical health and body's functionality. The cannabinoids also hold a secret for recovery from highly stressful events.

Dr. Irit Akirav, in the Department of Psychology at University of Haifa, Israel, published in *Frontiers in Behavioral Neuroscience* ("Targeting the endocannabinoid system to treat haunting traumatic memories"), documents that endocannabinoids help people get rid of the stress associated with traumatic experiences. Cannabinoid agonists that were administered shortly after exposure to stressful events prevented development of PTSD-like symptoms in rats (http://www.ncbi.nlm.nih.gov/pmc/articles/PMC3776936/).

The Endocannabinoid System and Anxiety

The endocannabinoid system is involved in the regulation of anxiety and fear responses. Evidence shows that anxiety is reduced by cannabinoids (http://www.ncbi.nlm.nih.gov/pubmed/24923339).

The endocannabinoid system balances the strengthening or maintenance of original memory and the establishment of new memory. This is important because this ability of the endocannabinoid system protects us from over-reacting to highly stressful events or situations.

Basically, the endocannabinoid system acts like a regulatory buffer system for our emotional responses to situations we encounter. Imagine the potential of this plant.

The Endocannabinoid System and Neural Pain

Neural pain occurs when neurons in the brain or peripheral nervous system become hypersensitive and start generating abnormal or prolonged impulses. Severe neural pain is often quite difficult to treat. More than 50 percent of patients report that medications and standard therapies aren't helpful for reducing the pain they experience or have undesirable side effects.

When allopathic medications are inadequate for whatever reason, cannabinoids are often effective! Cannabinoids are often more effective than opioids, pills, and other types of medications in relieving neural pain (http://www.ncbi.nlm.nih.gov/pmc/articles/PMC2430692/).

Cannabinoids impact normal inhibitory pathways and pathophysiological processes, thus reducing nociception, the processing of harmful stimuli in the Nervous System.

The Endocannabinoid System and Migraines

A migraine is an intense headache that is deeply associated with endocannabinoid deficiency. Imagine up until 1936, doctors prescribed cannabis to patients who were diagnosed with migraines. In fact, cannabis was more effective in relieving pain than aspirin, or some other painkillers.

The anti-migraine properties of cannabis have again been recognized (http://www.google.com/patents/US6630507—think vascular ischemic events of the central nervous system). Access to hemp-derived cannabidiol allows relief from migraine for many.

Sally Schutz, M.D. & Bayne Boyes, FCPA

The Endocannabinoid System and Chronic Vomiting Disorder

Chronic vomiting disorder is characterized by episodes of severe vomiting that have no exact cause. Cannabis has been used to treat nausea and vomiting for thousands of years, and the discovery of the endocannabinoid system created new ways of treating this condition.

Scientists discovered that impairment of the endocannabinoid system may cause vomiting, nausea, and even motion sickness. For example, in some studies, participants who experienced motion sickness had lower expression of CB1 receptors (http://www.ncbi.nlm.nih.gov/pubmed/24184696).

The Endocannabinoid System and Fibromyalgia

Fibromyalgia is characterized by pain sensation throughout the body. Stimulation of CB1 and CB2 receptors results in the relief of this elusive disease. As fibromyalgia generally doesn't have a cure, cannabis proves to be beneficial for helping tolerate symptoms of this disease due to its sedative, analgesic, and anti-inflammatory properties.

The Endocannabinoid System and Multiple Sclerosis

Historians report that cannabis was used in ancient China and Greece to relieve the symptoms linked with multiple sclerosis: muscle spasms and tremors. Contemporary studies confirm the effects of cannabis and the endocannabinoid system in multiple sclerosis and spasticities. Baker et al in *the Journal of the Federation of American Societies for Experimental Biology* http://www-.ncbi.nlm.nih.gov/pubmed/12849183) reported important evidence for the control of spasticity by the endocannabinoid system. They found that stimulation of CB1 and CB2 receptors has anti-inflammatory and neuroprotective potential because the endocannabinoid system controls the levels of neurodegeneration.

Neurodegeneration is a result of inflammatory "insults." Studies consistently point to cannabinoids slowing down the progression of neurodegenerative diseases.

The Endocannabinoid System and ALS

Manipulation of the endocannabinoid system and cannabis has beneficial effects on patients with ALS. Cannabinoids exert anti-inflammatory and anti-glutamatergic actions through activation of both CB1 and CB2 receptors (http://www.google.com/patents/US6630507).

The Endocannabinoid System and AIDS

Many diseases arise out of chronic inflammation, such as cancer, arthritis, brain injury, and AIDS. The inflammatory cytokines are activated by oxidative stress in which healthy cells are inhibited and destroyed.

Cannabinoids act as immuno-modulators. They interrupt the cytokine inflammatory action, thus preventing inflammation to result in tissue pathology. This slows down the progression of AIDS, which makes a person vulnerable to various diseases and infections.

The Endocannabinoid System and Cancer

The endocannabinoid system not only has the ability to inhibit and destroy cancer cells, but it also relieves the pain associated with cancer. Clinical trials that assess the effectiveness of cannabis extracts are ongoing (http://www.cancer.gov/about-cancer/treatment/cam/hp/cannabis-pdq).

The ECS also affects:

- sleep disorders
- glaucoma

- appetite
- memory
- much more

Other Possibilities that Involve the Endocannabinoid System

Throughout this chapter, you have had the opportunity to see many systems and parts of your body that are affected by the endocannabinoid system. But the truth is that this system affects and regulates our *entire* organism, which is why dysfunction and imbalance of cannabinoid receptors can lead to diseases.

What's next for Endocannabinoid Science?

The discovery of the endocannabinoid system could well be the single most important scientific medical discovery in the last century, or certainly at least one of the top five.

The ECS is the master control system of the body that regulates homeostasis and prevents disease and aging. Dr. David Allen a thoracic cardiovascular surgeon in a review of cannabis stated that "the majority of people in the United States have no idea of the remarkable, scientifically-proven medical benefits of cannabis. These cannabinoids are responsible for massive reductions in diabetes, stroke and myocardial scars."

Many cancers show significant responses to cannabinoids by:

1. Inhibition of growth of the tumor
2. Reduction in metastasis (blood and lymphatic spread of the cancer)
3. Inhibition of VEGF (vascular endothelial growth factor), which inhibits blood vessel growth into tumors (inhibiting vasculogenesis)
4. Induction of apoptosis-normal cell death that cancer cells are immune to

The Anti-Aging Miracles of Hemp-Derived CBD Oil

Dr. Allen goes on to report:

> Glucose and fatty metabolism, pain control and inflammation are all controlled by the ECS. There are many reports of patients with seizures that are unresponsive to all medicines except cannabis extracts. We are learning that even the sperm implantation into the ovum requires endocannabinoids for success. Humans have a hard time believing in things they can't see. Prior to the invention of the microscope, no medical schools taught sterile technique to their students because bacteria were unseen. (http://www.outwordmagazine.com/inside-outword/glbt-news/1266-survey-shows-low-acceptance-of-the-science-of-the-ecs-endocannabinoid-system)

Shockingly and unfortunately, according to the latest figures, only 13 percent of the medical schools in United States mention endocannabinoid science in their curriculum (http://www.outwordmagazine.com/inside-outword/glbt-news/1266-survey-shows-low-acceptance-of-the-science-of-the-ecs-endocannabinoid-system).

Overall, the ECS is a control system of body physiology that cannot be discounted or ignored. Medical schools can play down the importance of the ECS or even pretend it does not exist. Lewis reminds us that society and medical educators once questioned the significance of hand washing prior to surgical procedures because bacteria could not be seen by the naked eye. But the overwhelming anecdotal evidence, as well as the scientific research coming out of Israel and other parts of the world (U.S. included), cannot be dismissed.

People may not understand the complex science behind this natural herb, but they can understand that balancing the endocannabinoid system, the Master Control System is beneficial in many areas!

> People will demand hemp-derived CBD oil.
> It's from nature.

Sally Schutz, M.D. & Bayne Boyes, FCPA

It is safe.
It has been used for millennia.
It's not toxic.
It helps many health systems.
It assists the Master Control System!

CHAPTER 9

What is The Entourage Effect?

The "entourage effect" is a phrase that was introduced to cannabinoid science by Dr. Raphael Mechoulam and S. Ben-Shabat. The phrase is used to represent the endogenous cannabinoid molecular regulation route.

What Does It Really Mean?

Unlike most medicines and remedies used today, cannabis has a wide range of compounds. Scientists have identified 110 compounds out of which THC is the most notorious and controversial one because of its psychoactivity. However, it is widely accepted that the cannabis plant contains up to 480 different chemical compounds.

Among these 480 compounds, there are non-cannabinoid compounds that have certain regulatory effects. For example, terpenes are molecules that are responsible for the distinct smell of cannabis. (We are familiar with the distinct smells of pine and lemon, which are produced by their own terpenes.)

Terpenes are shown to block certain cannabinoid receptor sites in the brain while promoting cannabinoid binding in other receptor sites simultaneously. It is believed that terpenes affect different aspects of how our brain takes in CBD or THC (http://www.leafscience.com/2014/09/11/medical-marijuana-entourage-effect/).

Terpenes also have their own therapeutic benefits, which will be discussed below.

Although THC and CBD get the most attention from scientists who work in cannabinoid science, most scientists now agree that the different compounds in cannabis work together to produce a unique synergy of effects, which is known as the "entourage effect."

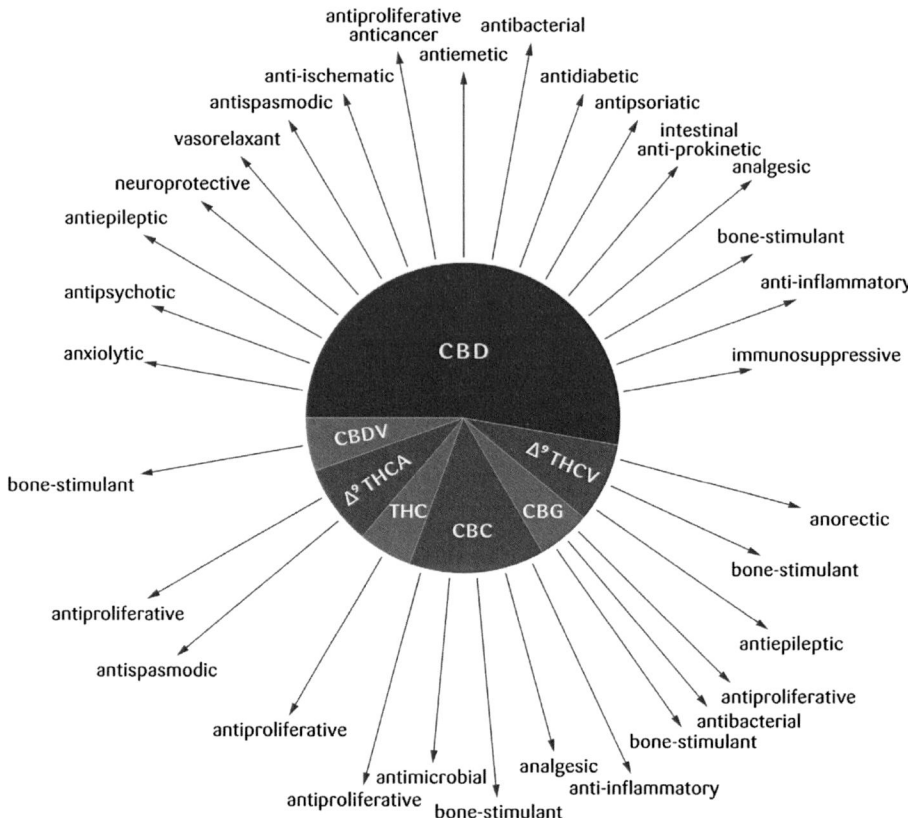

Cannabinoids and their benefits courtesy of BestCann.com

What are Terpenes?

As mentioned above, terpenes are compounds in cannabis that are responsible for the smell. They collaborate in an entourage effect but are also known for having their own therapeutic properties.

The Anti-Aging Miracles of Hemp-Derived CBD Oil

Terpenes aren't psychoactive compounds and can be used to successfully affect a wide array of symptoms. The number of terpenes in cannabis is huge, and the prominent ones include:

- Limonene—promotes weight loss, prevents and treats cancer, and is beneficial for bronchitis
- Myrcene—serves as an anti-inflammatory agent (it also works as a muscle relaxant and as a sedative)
- Linalool—treats liver cancer and helps modulate the motor movements
- Alpha Bisabolol—heals wounds and fights bacteria
- Delta 3 Carene—dries fluids like runny nose, menstrual flow, and tears
- Borneol—is analgesic (helps with insomnia, anti-septic, and bronchodilator)
- Alpha-pinene—serves as an anti-inflammatory agent
- Eucalyptol— serves as a cough suppressant and mouthwash
- Terpineol—is an antioxidant
- Caryophyllene—treats anxiety and depression
- Cineole—serves as an antibiotic and is antiviral and anti-inflammatory

A-PINENE	BETA CARYOPHYLLENE	MYRCENE	LIMONENE
ANTI-INFLAMMATORY BRONCHODILATOR AIDS MEMORY ANTI-BACTERIAL	ANTI-INFLAMMATORY ANALGESIC AIDS LINING OF DIGESTIVE TRACT	SEDATIVE SLEEP AID MUSCLE-RELAXANT	AIDS ACID REFLUX ANTI-ANXIETY ASSISTS MOOD
ALSO FOUND IN PINE NEEDLES	ALSO FOUND IN BLACK PEPPER	ALSO FOUND IN HOPS	ALSO FOUND IN CITRUS

Cannabis terpenes (courtesy of Kick Ass Energy)

Scientists are currently mapping and conducting studies on terpenes to fully understand their role in the overall benefits of cannabis.

What are Sterols?

Sterols are steroid alcohols, which is a subgroup of steroids and an important category of organic molecules. Sterols occur naturally in animals, plants, fungi, etc. This natural fatty plant substance impacts health in many areas including immunity and cardiovascular health.

Cannabis contains a variety of sterols including sitosterol.

SITOSTEROL

Web MD lists the known effects of sitosterol:

- regulating cholesterol
- protecting from cardiovascular diseases
- boosting the immune system
- preventing cancer

It also alleviated the symptoms of:

- arthritis
- psoriasis
- asthma
- lupus
- migraines
- fatigue
- HIV

The Anti-Aging Miracles of Hemp-Derived CBD Oil

Sitosterol

Image courtesy of Wikipedia

CAMPESTEROL

This type of sterol in cannabis helps other compounds to:

- balance cholesterol
- regulate the prostate

STIGMASTEROL

This type of sterol has a wide range of benefits including:

- an anti-osteoarthritic effect
- an apoptotic effect
- an antioxidant effect

This is not an exhaustive list of the anti-aging and health restorative compounds in cannabis. This is only a list to whet your appetite for the remarkable power of this amazing plant to bio-hack your body and protect you against aging.

CHAPTER 10

Mitochondrial Disease

EXISTING AS ORGANELLES or specialized compartments within the cell, mitochondria can be thought of as the "energy factory". By utilizing the oxygen breathed into the body and ingested food, mitochondria are able to generate the most basic energy unit of the human body known as ATP or adenosine triphosphate. From this angle it is easy to see how almost every organ and bodily process is touched by the effects and products of mitochondria. Without mitochondria, the heart, liver and brain will cease to function. Likewise, entire systems such as the endocrine and musculoskeletal systems will shut down. And without mitochondria, DNA and RNA, the very strands of life cannot be formed.

Imagine a world without sun. The climate would cool. Plants and animals would perish. Humanity and its constructs would follow. As apocalyptic as this may sound this is what it is like when the body develops mitochondrial disease. The cell no longer generates energy. It starves and dies. And much like the sun going dark, a catastrophic chain of events follows as organs collapse and different systems start to fail at once.

There are many symptoms to mitochondrial disease. Many of which we are all familiar with. However, the difficulty in properly diagnosing mitochondrial disease is to correctly attribute the symptoms observed with the correct condition. These symptoms include:

- Loss of motor control
- Muscle fatigue

- Muscle pain
- Gastrointestinal disorders
- Cardiac disease
- Liver disease
- Diabetes
- Developmental delays & poor growth
- Respiratory complications
- Seizures
- Susceptibility to disease

In 2014 a team of researchers studied the effects of the endocannabinoid system (ECS) on mitochondrial function. The study revealed that the ECS modulates mitochondria function. By increasing oxidative phosphorylation and energy generation, the cannabinoid receptors, CB1 and CB2, have been shown to improve the function and capacity of mitochondria when activated[13]. The best thing is that this was not an isolated incident. Throughout the years, multiple studies have been conducted to delve into function of mitochondria while under the influence of cannabinoids. The results of these experiments were eye-opening to say the least.

When introduced to rodents, cannabidiol (CBD) has been shown to cause a significant increase in the function of mitochondria[14]. A similar study echoed these results when two cannabinoids, both of which were non-psychoactive, were shown to have a positive effect in mitochondrial

---

13 Lipina, C., Irving, A.J., and Hundal, H.S. (2014, July 1). Mitochondria: a possible nexus for the regulation of energy homeostasis by the endocannabinoid system? American Journal of Physiology. Endocrinology and Metabolism, 307(1). Retrieved from http://www.ncbi.nlm.nih.gov/pubmed/24801388. - See more at: http://medicalmarijuanainc.com/mitochondrial-disease-medical-marijuana-research/#sthash.9kZU3w50.dpuf

14 Bilkei-Gorzo, A. (2012, October 29). The endocannabinoid system in normal and pathological brain ageing. Philosophical Transactions of the Royal Society, B, 367(1607). Retrieved from http://rstb.royalsocietypublishing.org/content/367/1607/3326.abstract?sid=20cf2c23-e4fd-49e3-9398-ec8be2e00226. - See more at: http://medicalmarijuanainc.com/mitochondrial-disease-medical-marijuana-research/#sthash.9kZU3w50.dpuf

activity[15]. In 2015, researchers treated a cell whose mitochondrial parameters were intentionally changed with cannabinoids. They found that not only did the parameters revert back to its normal range, but also increase the potential of the mitochondrial membrane[16].

mTOR Pathways

Mitochondria may very well be the "energy factory" of the cell. However, left to its own devices it will continuously produce energy until it or the cell burns out. Think of it like a firehose without a nozzle. It will continuously spurt water at high pressure without a care in the world. What it needs is a nozzle. It needs to be controlled and regulated. And, that's why we have the mTOR pathway.

It stands for mechanistic target or rapamycin, and is primarily a signaling pathway. Operating both inside and out of the cell, the mTOR pathway is most closely associated with the regulation of metabolism, but it also has secondary effects on growth, proliferation and survival. Triggered by any number of events ranging from insulin fluctuations, cancer formation and even the activation of the immune system. If your body needs energy to move, grow, heal, and fight you can be sure that it will be utilizing the mTOR pathway to do so.

Using the multiprotein complexes known as mTORC1 and mTORC2, the pathway can prompt different responses. mTORC1 elicits a more direct response as it controls the production of proteins and lipids, but it also

---

15 Silvestri, C., Paris, D., Martella, A., Melck, D., Guadagnino, I., Cawthorne, M., Motta, A., and Di Marzo, V. (2015, June). Two non-psychoactive cannabinoids reduce intracellular lipid levels and inhibit hepatosteatosis. Journal of Hepatology, 62(6), 1382-90. - See more at: http://medicalmarijuanainc.com/mitochondrial-disease-medical-marijuana-research/#sthash.9kZU3w50.dpuf

16 Lu, Y., and Anderson, H.D. (2015, June). 6B.09: Effect of Cannabinoid Receptor Activation on Aberrant Mitochondrial Bioenergetics in Hypertrophied Cardiac Myocytes. Journal of Hypertension. 33. Retrieved from http://www.ncbi.nlm.nih.gov/pubmed/26102932. - See more at: http://medicalmarijuanainc.com/mitochondrial-disease-medical-marijuana-research/#sthash.9kZU3w50.dpuf

sets the limits on the catabolic processes of the cell and body. It accomplishes this by reacting to the signals released by oxygen and amino acid activity, growth factors and by monitoring the energy level of the body.

mTORC2 on the other hand, plays more of a backseat role. It is less direct in its approach and merely influences processes such as cytoskeletal organization, survival, metabolic output and proliferation.

mTOR does have a darkside however. Yes, it has been associated with energy supply, growth and survival, but it studies have also linked it with the development of cancers and diseases. Several forms of cancer have been connected with the abnormal activity of the mTOR pathway[17]. Likewise, over-activity of the pathway has shown to increase resistance to therapies for various types of cancers. In 2006, a team of researchers showed that in patients who are diabetic, obese, depressed or suffer from forms of cancer[18] have highly compromised mTOR pathways. To combat this, researchers and scientists have theorized that since mTOR targets rapamycin, then by reversing the process, and reintroduce rapamycin, they can inhibit the pathway and have a significant impact on cancer treatment[19].

CBD and the mTOR pathway

The two-faced nature mTOR has given it a questionable reputation. On one hand we depend on it to regulate metabolism, on the other hand it can cause cancer and disease. It seems that the line between the two worlds is razor thin. How then can we keep it in our lives without living in constant fear of our health. Studies conducted throughout the last decade may show a glimmer of hope in CBD. A team of researchers introduced CBD to breast cancer cells in 2011 leading to the inhibition of the mTOR

---

[17] Myers AP and Cantley LC: Targeting a common collaborator in cancer development. Sci Transl Med. 2:48ps452010

[18] McCubrey JA, Steelman LS, Franklin RA, et al: Targeting the RAF/MEK/ERK, PI3K/AKT and p53 pathways in hematopoietic drug resistance. Adv Enzyme Regul. 47:64–103. 2007

[19] Beevers CS, Li F, Liu L, Huang S (2006). "Curcumin inhibits the mammalian target of rapamycin-mediated signaling pathways in cancer cells". Int J Cancer 119 (4): 757–64. doi:10.1002/ijc.21932. PMID 16550606

pathway and killing the cancer cells20. CBD is thought to have a neuroprotective effect on cells which was shown in action when researchers, using cocaine, induced seizures in mice. When CBD was introduced, the seizures decreased. In comparison, the seizures only got worse when rapamycin was introduced. This led the team to believe that by activating the mTOR pathway, CBD has the ability to generate a neuroprotective effect21.

On a separate but not unrelated note, a study in schizophrenic patients may have revealed another CBD-mTOR connection. Schizophrenia is thought to be the result of an overstimulated dopamine receptor. It is hypothesized that the activity in the dopamine receptor can be decreased by controlling the downstream signaling of the mTOR pathway through the introduction of CBD22.

---

20 hrivastava A, Kuzontkoski PM, Groopman JE, Prasad A. Cannabidiol induces programmed cell death in breast cancer cells by coordinating the cross-talk between apoptosis and autophagy. Mol Cancer Ther 2011; 10:

21 Gobira PH, et al. Cannabidiol, a Cannabis sativa constituent, inhibits cocaine-induced seizures in mice: Possible role of the mTOR pathway and reduction in glutamate release. Neurotoxicity. 2015; 50: 116-21. http://www.ncbi.nlm.nih.gov/pubmed/26283212

22 Renard J, et al. Cannabidiol counteracts amphetamine-induced neuronal and behavioural sensitization of the mesolimbic dopamine pathway through a novel mTOR/p70S6 kinase signaling pathway. The Journal of Neuroscience. 2016; 36(18): 5160-5169. http://www.jneurosci.org/content/36/18/5160.short

CHAPTER 11

CBD Oil

CBD OIL is the easy to pronounce and common term for cannabidiol oil. Cannabidiol is defined as a natural component of cannabis. Throughout this chapter, we're going to see what CBD oil is and what amazing benefits it has.

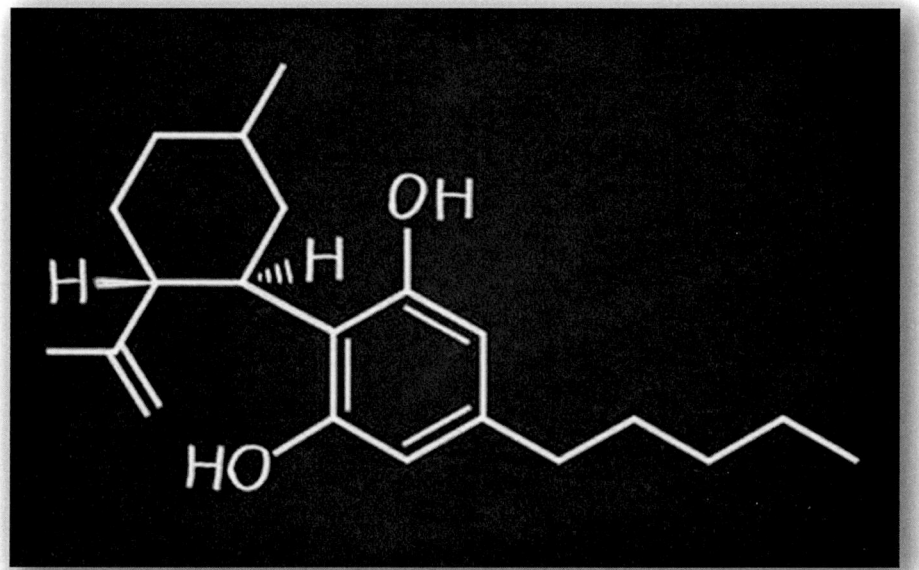

Image courtesy of Makaule: Shutterstock.com

CBD Oil—Basics

The oil is made of flowers, leaves, and stalks of cannabis. This is actually the most important difference between the CBD oil and "regular" hemp oil, which is primarily made of the seeds of the plant (http://www.chronictherapy.co/hemp-oil-vs-cbd-oil-whats-the-difference-2/).

CANNABIDIOL—CBD

CBD is gaining popularity in people seeking alternative health modalities because it can help alleviate various symptoms. For example:

- It has known apoptotic effects: the death of cells that occurs as a normal and regulated part of an organism's growth or development.
- It has natural analgesic properties.
- It controls seizures in many otherwise uncontrollable epileptics.
- It controls and eliminates intractable nausea arising from chemotherapy.
- It has anti-inflammatory properties.
- It regulates mood disorders of many types (in fact, the U.S. patent of 2003 #6630507 states it is anxiolytic).

CBG—Cannabigerol

While we're getting to know CBD and all its benefits, it's important to mention CBG, which is, in fact, CBD's precursor. CBG is short for *Cannabigerol*, and it is a non-psychoactive cannabinoid that is found in marijuana and hemp. CBG like CBD is found in higher concentrations in hemp. CBG is also highly beneficial in treating a variety of different diseases, including inflammatory bowel disease (IBD). IBD is considered to be an "incurable" disease that affects millions of people around the world. A study conducted by Francesca Borrelli from the Department of Pharmacy at the University of Naples Federico II demonstrated that CBG can have beneficial effects on patients who suffer from IBD (*http://www.researchgate.net/profile/Francesca_Borrelli/publication/26751588_Cannabidiol_a_safe_and_non-psychotropic_ingredient_of_the_marijuana_plant_Cannabis_sativa_is_protective_in_a_murine_model_of_colitis/links/02e7e51c98702822cf000000.pdf*).

The Anti-Aging Miracles of Hemp-Derived CBD Oil

CBD Oil is Not Psychoactive

Some people worry that CBD oil will "get them high" since it's made of cannabis. This is not the case because hemp-derived CBD oil by definition contains an insignificant amount of THC, the substance that is psychoactive. Thus, we say CBD oil is non-psychoactive.

Throughout this book, we have already established THC is the notorious and psychoactive component of marijuana. However, CBD does NOT have any psychoactive properties. *Why?* CBD doesn't act on the same receptors or pathways as THC. Thus CBD oil with less than 0.3% THC is not psychoactive.

In fact, the patent on cannabidiol (US6630507) indicates that CBD oil is safe to use. Research has shown that taking 100 times the normal dose is not lethal. It has even been used in children suffering from intractable epilepsy. Some children diagnosed with tumors, cancer, and epilepsy have benefited from taking this oil without experiencing any known harmful side effects.

The Legal Status of CBD Oil

Legal CBD oil is made from agricultural hemp because it has a THC level lower than 3%. However, under Federal law, it is still not legal to grow agricultural hemp in the United States, which is why hemp products are imported. However, CBD oil made from agricultural hemp is legal to import, purchase, and use across the United States.

In other countries, the law is more complex, and the best way to find out whether you can purchase CBD oil legally is to research and become informed about the laws in your country.

CHAPTER 12

Why Are Cannabinoids Better than Prescription Drugs for Pain, Anxiety, and Sleep?

LET'S REVIEW THIS one issue at a time.

Pain

Pain Medications have side effects.

Advil is touted as relief that "doesn't get any better than this."

But what about Advil's side effects? Have you read the insert? "It can cause severe allergic reaction, stomach bleeding. It can cause blood pressure to rise and puts stress on the heart and kidneys."

According to webmd.com, Advil "can even increase the risk for heart attack or stroke, especially in higher doses."

Stronger pain medication known as the opioid drugs, including Codeine, Dilaudid, Oxycontin and Percocet, have other nasty side effects: addiction, constipation, drowsiness, and especially *overdose*.

Taking pain medication with sleeping pills, antihistamines, or antidepressants can be even more dangerous.

The Anti-Aging Miracles of Hemp-Derived CBD Oil

IBUPROFEN 2 Tablets

Image courtesy of Iodine.com

In 2014, Dr. Nora Volkow, chair of the NIDA, a division of the NIH, asserted at the Senate Caucus on International Narcotics Control:

> The abuse of and addiction to opioids such as heroin, morphine, and prescription pain relievers is a serious global problem that affects the health, social, and economic welfare of all societies. It is estimated that between 26.4 million and 36 million people abuse opioids worldwide [1] with an estimated 2.1 million people in the United States suffering from substance use disorders related to prescription opioid pain relievers in 2012 and an estimated 467,000 addicted to heroin.

ANXIETY

How about tranquilizers and anti-anxiety meds? We all know someone taking Xanax, Valium or Ativan. Chronic use of benzodiazepines (anti-anxiety medications) are associated with depression. Let's look at the drug insert for Valium:

ADVERSE REACTIONS

Side effects most commonly reported were drowsiness, fatigue, muscle weakness, and ataxia. The following have also been reported:

Central Nervous System: confusion, depression, dysarthria, headache, slurred speech, tremor, vertigo

Gastrointestinal System: constipation, nausea, gastrointestinal disturbances

Special Senses: blurred vision, diplopia, dizziness

Cardiovascular System: hypotension

Psychiatric and Paradoxical Reactions: stimulation, restlessness, acute hyperexcited states, anxiety, agitation, aggressiveness, irritability, rage, hallucinations, psychoses, delusions, increased muscle spasticity, insomnia, sleep disturbances, and nightmares. Inappropriate behavior and other adverse behavioral effects have been reported when using benzodiazepines. Should these occur, use of the drug should be discontinued. They are more likely to occur in children and in the elderly.

Urogenital System: incontinence, changes in libido, urinary retention

Skin and Appendages: skin reactions

Laboratories: elevated transaminases and alkaline phosphatase

Other: changes in salivation, including dry mouth, hypersalivation

Figure 3: Drug insert for Valium

SLEEP

Sleep is critical to good health—its restorative, but in fact 60 million Americans are affected adversely by insomnia yearly. Gayle Greene, author of *Insomniac*, writes, "Sleep is the fuel of life. It's nourishing; it's restorative. And when you are deprived of it, you are really deprived of a basic kind of sustenance."

So, what are the side effects of the major sleeping pills like Lunesta, Sonata, Ambien and Halcion?

The side effects of these sleep pharmaceuticals include:

- burning or tingling in the hands, arm, feet, or legs
- changes in appetite
- constipation
- diarrhea
- dizziness & difficulty keeping balance
- Impairment the next day and daytime drowsiness
- dry mouth or throat
- gas
- headache
- heartburn
- weakness
- unusual dreams

SAFETY:
Cannabis stimulates endocannabinoid receptors and improves the function of the entire endocannabinoid system. We cannot help but show a part of the US government patent 6630507, which in no uncertain terms describes cannabinoids as safe! Here is an extract from the patent, "Previous studies have also indicated that cannabidiol is not toxic, even when chronically administered to humans or given in large acute doses (700 mg/day)."

Sally Schutz, M.D. & Bayne Boyes, FCPA

Cannabinoids as antioxidants and neuroprotectants
US 6630507 B1

ABSTRACT

Cannabinoids have been found to have antioxidant properties, unrelated to NMDA receptor antagonism. This new found property makes cannabinoids useful in the treatment and prophylaxis of wide variety of oxidation associated diseases, such as ischemic, age-related, inflammatory and autoimmune diseases. The cannabinoids are found to have particular application as neuroprotectants, for example in limiting neurological damage following ischemic insults, such as stroke and trauma, or in the treatment of neurodegenerative diseases, such as Alzheimer's disease, Parkinson's disease and HIV dementia. Nonpsychoactive cannabinoids, such as cannabidiol, are particularly advantageous to use because they avoid toxicity that is encountered with psychoactive cannabinoids at high doses useful in the method of the present invention. A particular disclosed class of cannabinoids useful as neuroprotective antioxidants is formula (I) wherein the R group is independently selected from the group consisting of H, CH_3, and $COCH_3$.

Publication number	US6630507 B1
Publication type	Grant
Application number	US 09/674,028
PCT number	PCT/US1999/008769
Publication date	Oct 7, 2003
Filing date	Apr 21, 1999
Priority date	Apr 21, 1998
Fee status	Paid
Also published as	CA2329626A1, 4 More »
Inventors	Aidan J. Hampson, Julius Axelrod, Maurizio Grimaldi
Original Assignee	The United States Of America As Represented By The Department Of Health And Human Services
Export Citation	BiBTeX, EndNote, RefMan

Patent Citations (22), Non-Patent Citations (29), Referenced by (27), Classifications (16), Legal Events (5)
External Links: USPTO, USPTO Assignment, Espacenet

SUMMARY OF THE INVENTION

It is an object of this invention to provide a new class of antioxidant drugs, that have particular application as neuroprotectants, although they are generally useful in the treatment of many oxidation associated diseases.

Yet another object of the invention is to provide a subset of such drugs that can be substantially free of psychoactive or psychotoxic effects, are substantially non-toxic even at very high doses, and have good tissue penetration, for example crossing the blood brain barrier.

It has surprisingly been found that cannabidiol and other cannabinoids can function as neuroprotectants, even though they lack NMDA receptor antagonist activity. This discovery was made possible because of the inventor's recognition of a previously unanticipated antioxidant property of the cannabinoids in general (and cannabidiol in particular) that functions completely independently of antagonism at the NMDA, AMPA and kainate receptors. Hence the present invention includes methods of preventing or treating diseases caused by oxidative stress, such as neuronal hypoxia, by administering a prophylactic or therapeutically effective amount of a cannabinoid to a subject who has a disease caused by oxidative stress.

Image Credit: Booth and Garion/ Science Source - composite image of a Kirlian photograph of Cannabis sativa.

The Anti-Aging Miracles of Hemp-Derived CBD Oil

Prescription drugs have the opposite effect. While they often help various symptoms for which they were designed and formulated, they can simultaneously adversely affect the function of other organs and systems producing serious sometimes life threatening side effects. We all see the advertisements on TV and in magazines—how often do they mention really serious side effects, sometimes even including death?

Conclusion

WE WOULD LIKE to finish with a brief mention of the fact that we are embarking on a critical time in the evolution of cannabis in the United States. As we have discussed, hemp-derived cannabidiol is safe; it is legal; it is effective in the alleviation of a wide variety of conditions.

Moreover, imagine its usefulness in the healthy individual to biohack and maintain a healthy endocannabinoid system—to bulletproof the master control system that controls homeostasis in the body. Imagine how a regular routine of non-psychoactive cannabinoid compounds could protect:

- your brain
- your bones
- your immune system
- your cytokine (inflammatory) system
- your mood
- your gut

And the list is growing...

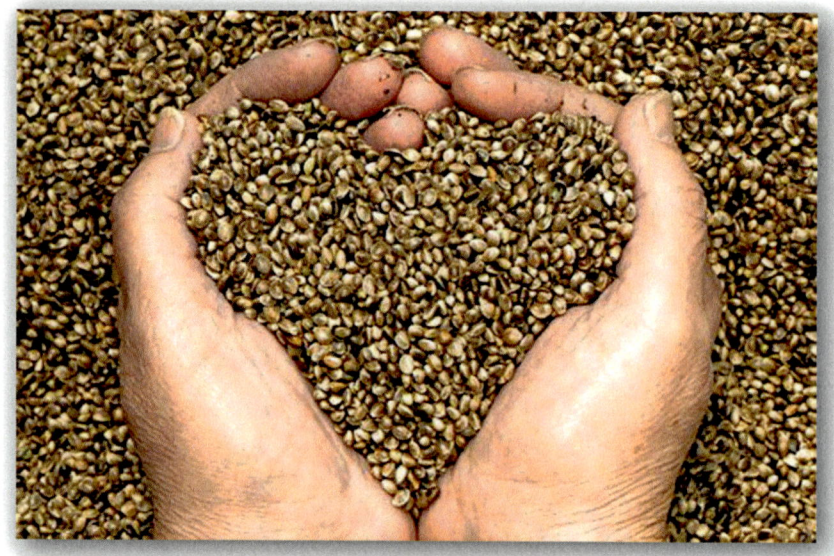

courtesy of Jade: shutterstock.com

Imagine balancing the *major control system* of the body.

Imagine reducing stress.

Isn't that what everyone wants?

Something that will protect our health and well-being?

A natural plant that balances the *master control system* of the body, the ECS.

The status of cannabis is evolving, and you, by reading this book, have contributed to its universal intelligence.

The Anti-Aging Miracles of Hemp-Derived CBD Oil

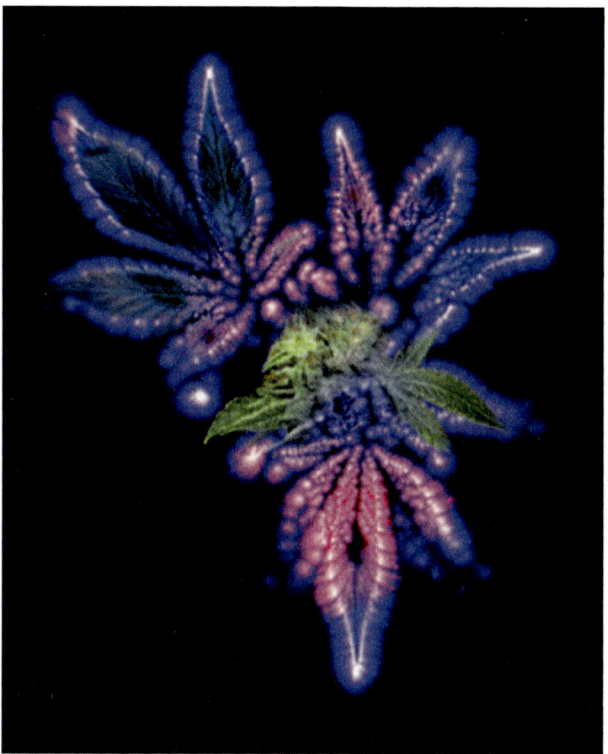

Image Courtesy of Booth and Garion/ Science Source – composite image of a Kirlian photograph of Cannabis sativa.

And for that, we personally thank you.

If you like this book, kindly rate and review it on Facebook/TheAntiAgingMiracles.

Made in the USA
San Bernardino, CA
17 August 2017